# Gender dysphoria

Des mêmes auteurs

**By Gérard and Nicole Delépine**

*Dysphorie de genre*, Fauves, 2023.

*Hystérie vaccinale. Gardasil et cancer: un paradoxe, Fauves, 2018 ; new revised and expanded edition*, Fauves, 2023.

*Les enfants sacrifiés du Covid. Isolement, masques et vaccins*, Fauves, 2022.

*Autopsie d'un confinement aveugle*, Fauves, 2020.

*Gardasil (english)* Fauves, 2019.

*Médicaments anti-cancer peu efficaces, souvent toxiques et hors de prix*, Michalon, 2017.

*Soigner et obéir. Premières mesures urgentes pour éviter le naufrage*, Fauves, 2016.

*Cancer. Les bonnes questions à poser à votre médecin*, Michalon, 2016.

**By Nicole Delépine**

*Neuf petits lits sur le trottoir*, Fauves, 2014.

*Le cancer, un fléau qui rapporte*, Michalon, 2013.

*La face cachée des médicaments*, Michalon, 2011.

*Ma liberté de soigner*, Michalon, 2005.

*Neuf petits lits au fond du couloir*, Michalon, 2000.

website Docteur Nicole Delépine – Site Officiel du Docteur Nicole Delépine, Pédiatre, Oncologie (nicoledelepine.fr) Nicole Delepine ses publications médicales sur ses travaux pour la lutte contre le cancer)


9, rue de l'École-Polytechnique – 75005 Paris
www.fauves-editions.fr
ISBN : 979-10-302-0518-3

Nicole & Gérard Delépine

# Gender dysphoria

## Hormones, surgery, transformations…
## Risks and pitfalls of gender transition in children and teenagers

FAUVES
ÉDITIONS

To all the children of the world, so that they can live their childhood freely and safely, so that their imagination and creativity are not blocked by age- non appropriate interventions.

To older people who have questions about their "gender" to be able to think about it, freely with enough medical information that allows for truly informed consent.

Our approach is purely medical and benevolent for everyone, especially the transitioners, who are too often victims of misinformation and manipulation, so that they do not become hostages of societal, academic and/or financial lobbies, while the trans market achieves fabulous sums reaching billions of dollars.

# Introduction
# No, sex is not a space-sex amusement park![1][2]

Why this book on gender theory now, when it has been spreading in France for several decades and most notably in the state education system since 2014?
It is high time that families and teachers were informed about the danger posed to children by the information they are given at school (and elsewhere) at an age when they are incapable in every respect (intellectually, emotionally, psychologically) of weighing up its effects and being able to choose their orientation.
Their protection is, to our mind, a categorical imperative because we, as children's doctors, paediatricians and surgeons, have direct experience of the fragility of boys and girls and of the importance of choosing the right words (when giving a diagnosis or treatment, for example) to explain without causing hurt or loss of trust.

1. https://actionetdemocratie.com/education-a-la-sexualite/
2. The website approved by Santé Publique France reads: "*Le sexe, c'est comme un parc d'attractions (masturbatrain, space-sex).*"

It is an artform that we have been trying to develop over the decades with varying degrees of effectiveness, success and failure. Simply saying "*it's going to be all right, it'll pass*" or "*there are worse things*" can be outrageous to the young patient who fears that his/her pain has not been understood.

The appearance on a government website aimed at children of these cold statements and advice on sexuality has sent shivers through us as parents, grandparents and doctors. Social media influencers are (quite rightly) accused of unsettling our youngsters, but it is time to sound the alarm when the ministry and other government or government-approved agencies behave similarly.
Our concern with sites aimed at minors under state guardianship has prompted us to write this book. The strength of the propaganda and the reactions to this intrusion into people's lives are such that it could stretch to several volumes, but we shall confine ourselves to exploring a few fundamental points, systematically sourced medical facts in the main, to give everyone the opportunity to learn for themselves.

The issue is making headlines in the media now that male-born transgender athletes are seeking to take part in women's events at the 2024 Olympic Games, and the Minister for Sport, when questioned about her decision, remains vague and passes the buck to the federations. Let us remind ourselves that gender theory is a political and ideological concept, not a medical one, unlike sex which is a biological reality.

**"Sex is not an opinion, it's an anthropological fact"[3]**
A marginal phenomenon in terms of the number of people actually affected in France (a few thousand), its infiltration into all spheres of influence - political, cultural and educational – has turned a feeling, a respectable individual choice into an ideological battle that is destabilising education and culture and can no longer be ignored. You can change your gender, but not your sex, says Emeritus Professor of Medical Genetics Claudine Junien, along with many others. We can imagine the practical consequences of this statement in everyone's life.
Feelings are not an anthropological fact, unlike the height, heart weight, lung volume and muscle mass of individuals with XY chromosomes, which remain much greater than those born XX and thus distort the results of sporting events, particularly at the highest level, when self-declared transgender women (born male and therefore XY) compete with female-born athletes.
Sixty years of feminist struggles and hard-won rights are threatened by this Trojan horse of men claiming to be women in sporting events, at school, and in places formerly reserved for women by birth (dormitories, changing rooms, toilets). The Olympic Games quintessentially. It stands to reason that no trans person who has become a man but has retained the physical capacities associated with their XX chromosomes will ever try to compete with boys, the latter obviously having no chance of beating them, as we shall explore later.
First-wave feminists are beginning to tear their hair out

3. JO 2024 : « Les athlètes femmes seront-elles remplacées par des hommes ? » – IREF Europe FR.

at the destruction of their decades-long struggle.[4]
The freedom of everyone to be homosexual, transgender, bisexual or any other variation of the concept posed no problem until a minority wanted to impose its model and gain power at all levels of society. This sectarian minority, rejected by others who wish to live their lives in peace, decided to impose transgenderism as the "*new normal*". And it is this that we cannot accept.
It is time for us all to open our eyes to what is no longer a marginal phenomenon, but a systemic trend that is putting at risk the mental health of our children and future generations.
We will therefore try to set out here as factually as possible what gender theory is and what its practical consequences are for young people in particular.
The aim of this little book is to provide a few tools and some answers for distraught families who suddenly discover that their 12-year-old daughter wants to take male hormones (available on the Internet) and bandage her breasts, or even have them removed by unscrupulous surgeons who are often driven by financial interests, thereby compromising permanently her ability to breastfeed her child, should she decide years later to become "herself" again.

4. *"Mrs Elisabeth Borne, feminists, we are concerned about what is becoming of Family Planning". (marianne.net). "As feminists, we are fighting for the abolition of gender stereotypes and not for their reinforcement as advocated by transactivism. We believe that what connects us all is our sex, not a penchant for couture, pink and Barbie dolls. We believe that men should have the right to cry in public, wear skirts and do gymnastics without being insulted as "pussies" or "faggots". We think we need to change mentalities rather than bodies. If we abolish these stereotypes, the need for transitions will be much less."*

# 1.
# A brief historical overview of "gender theory"

It is now a given in the media that those who regard a man as a man and a woman as a woman are conservative, has-been "*old-fashioned, outdated, reactionary*". Because, as Health Minister Agnès Buzyn explained on the LCP Channel on 24 September 2019, "*a grandmother can be a father…*".

**Where does "gender theory" come from?**

Discussion about gender issues only really started at the turn of the 20th century, at a time of advances in medicine[5]. Literature has always depicted people who feel they are of a different sex to the one they were born with. In villages, meanwhile, the matter was hushed up and anomalies accepted. The advent of endocrinology, coupled with the growth of Big Pharma, led to the belief that biology could solve the problem and deliver a client base.

5. Dysphorie de GENRE – Le mirage de la TRANSITION (odysee.com).

Attempts at a psychoanalytical explanation then followed. In Canada, doctors began to treat these children through psychotherapy, thinking that something else lay behind the malaise. In fact, during their adolescence, these children followed through with their gender transition in fewer than 15 % of cases. By and large, these children were already doing better on reaching adulthood, more often than not coming to terms with and identifying as homosexual.

**1949 – Kinsey, pioneer of the sexualisation of children**

The beginnings of gender theory appear to date back to 1949, when Dr Alfred Kinsey, professor of entomology and zoology[6], published his reports on sexuality in the USA, setting himself up as the "*father of the sexual revolution*". In his book *Sexual Behavior in the Human Male* (Table 34 of which is reproduced in the Annex[7]), he describes, among other things, repeated rapes of children and infants, followed, according to him, by orgasms, thus providing a "scientific" alibi for paedophilia.

Until her death, Dr Judith Reisman[8] fought relentlessly to denounce the biased selection of participants in the

6. Le Dr Alfred Kinsey, père de la « théorie du genre » : torture, pédophilie sur les nourrissons au nom de la science ! (lemediaen442.fr)

7. Pages 175-180.

8. Author of *Kinsey, Sex and Fraud : The Indoctrination of a People*, Lafayette, Huntington House, 1990.

Soft Porn Plays Hardball : Its Tragic Effects on Women, Children and the Family, Lafayette, Huntington House, 1991, "Kinsey : Crimes & Consequences : The Red Queen and the Grand Scheme", Crestwood, The Institute for Media Education, 1998, *Kinsey's Attic : The Shocking Story of How One Man's Sexual Pathology Changed the World*, Cumberland House, 2006, *Sexual Sabotage : How One Mad Scientist Unleashed a Plague of Corruption and Contagion on America*, Washington, WND Books, 2010.

study and the false claims of Alfred Kinsey whose conduct, in her view, was not of a neutral scientist, but of a champion of a pleasure-based sexuality with no limits. She refutes his claims in an attempt to save children from the perverted adults who use Alfred Kinsey's writings to try to sexualise them from birth. She showed that Alfred Kinsey had based his work in part on the testimony of a former Nazi officer turned cemetery caretaker, Fritz von Balluseck, who had raped hundreds of children. How could these babies have had orgasms and how could this have been observed? One 4-year-old child is said to have had 26 orgasms in 24 hours!

In her documentary Alfred Kinsey: pédophilie et révolution sexuelle, Marion Sigaut also shows that the reports were faked and were written by paedophiles, including Alfred Kinsey himself[9]. What's most astounding is that in 2019 Kinsey was honoured by Indiana University which erected a statue of him on the 75th anniversary of the Institute that bears his name. To mark the occasion, the Institute's President Pamela Whitten said: "*Around the nation and around the world, the Kinsey Institute is the trusted source for information on critical issues in human sexuality, relationships, gender and reproduction*".

That same year, in June 2019, Alfred Kinsey was one of the inaugural fifty American "pioneers, trailblazers and heroes" inducted on the National LGBTQ Wall of Honor within the Stonewall National Monument (SNM) in New York City, a monument dedicated to LGBTQ+ rights and history[10], a clear demonstration of the close

9. *Kinsey: Pedophilia and the Sexual Revolution, American report on paedophilia.*

10. Donde Vamos: "A tribute to Alfred Kinsey, the paedophile criminal who used child rape to try and provide a basis for his theory of child sexuality".

link between sex education, paedophilia and the LGBTQ+ lobby[11].

**1955 – John Money defines gender**

New Zealand sexologist and psychologist John Money, a specialist in hermaphroditism at Johns Hopkins University in the USA, after studying cases of intersex born children[12], defined gender in 1955 as the sexual conduct we choose to adopt, irrespective of our sex at birth.

***Catastrophic medical experiment on twins[13]***

In 1966, he founded the Gender Identity Clinic at John Hopkins University, the first of its kind in the United States, and launched an extensive research programme on the psychohormonal treatment of paraphilias and on "sex reassignment".

His first gender theory experiment ended in disaster with a set of twins born as boys. The parents of the eight-month-old twins wanted to have them circumcised, but the penis of one twin, Bruce, was burned as a result of electrical cauterisation. John Money leapt at the opportunity, hoping to demonstrate that biological sex was a sham, and suggested that the desperate parents raise Bruce as a girl, without ever revealing his birth sex. The parents acquiesced.

11. https://news.iu.edu/stories/2022/09/iub/releases/09-alfred-kinsey-sculpture.html

12. "Intersexuality or hermaphroditism: an individual who is born with both male and female attributes, either genetically (chromosomal anomaly) or as a result of a tumour (adrenal or sex gland tumour)" Cuenot et Rostand, Introduction à la génétique (1936).

13. https://www.lefigaro.fr/actualite-france/2014/01/31/01016-20140131ARTFIG00151-theorie-du-genre-comment-la-premiere-experimentation-a-mal-tourne.php

Bruce-Brenda was given hormones, had his testicles removed and was raised as a girl, complete with dresses and dolls. Everything seemingly went well during childhood, so much so that Money, believing he had succeeded, published numerous articles in praise of his "discovery" and even a book in 1972[14] in which he asserted that upbringing, and not one's sex at birth, determines whether one is male or female.

Reality, however, dramatically reared its ugly head. As a teenager, Brenda's voice broke and she found herself attracted to girls. Her parents owned up to the deception. She had the courage and strength of character to stop taking her female hormones and was given testosterone, the male hormone. *From then on, Brenda reverted to being a man, David, who had a surgically recreated penis and his breasts removed. He even married a woman at the age of 24. However, this extraordinary experience left the twins with irreparable damage. Brian committed suicide in 2002 and David in May 2004*".

**Links between transgenderism and paedophilia**

John Money's gender ideology led him to regard paedophilia as normal sexual behaviour : he believed that "affectional paedophilia" was based on love, not sex, and that affectional paedophilia was caused by an excess of parental love that became erotic, and was therefore not a behavioural disorder.

14. Man & Woman, Boy & Girl : The Differentiation and Dimorphism of Gender Identity from Conception to Maturity. A Mentor Book. Johns Hopkins paperback : Science.

John Money's interview with *Paidika*, a notorious paedophile magazine, in the spring of 1991[15] is clear: "*If I were to see the case of a boy aged 10 or 11 who's intensely attracted to a man in his twenties or thirties, if the relationship is totally mutual... then I would not call it pathological in any way*".

**1968 – Sexual revolution and promotion of paedophilia in the name of freedom**

On the set of prime-time talk show *Apostrophes* in April 1982[16], Daniel Cohn-Bendit declared: "*A child's sexuality is a fantastic thing. You have to be honest and sincere. I used to work with four-to-six-year-olds. When a little, five-year-old girl starts undressing you, it's amazing, it's an incredibly erotic game*".

As put more simply by the popular French singer Claude François, who had a daughter with a Belgian fan aged 14[17] at the time, "*I like girls until they're 17 or 18, then I start to distrust them.*"[18]

Since then, there have been calls from many prominent "sixty-eighter" writers and political activists for the law to make paedophilia legal.

On 26 January 1977, Jean-Paul Sartre, Roland Barthes, Simone de Beauvoir, Gilles and Fanny Deleuze, Francis Ponge, Philippe Sollers, Jack Lang, Bernard Kouchner,

15. Joseph Geraci and Donald Mader: "Interview: John Money" (p. 2-13) *Paidika,* Number 7, Spring 1991.

16. https://www.radiofrance.fr/franceculture/quand-des-intellectuels-francais-defendaient-la-pedophilie-2026242

17. https://www.facebook.com/watch/?v=1841016959305685

18. https://www.gala.fr/l_actu/news_de_stars/jaime-les-filles-jusqua-17-18-ans-la-petite-phrase-de-claude-francois-qui-devoile-lautre-facette-du-chanteur_412292

Louis Aragon, Gabriel Matzneff, André Glucksmann, François Châtelet, Guy Hocquenghem and a total of 69 French intellectuals, from Félix Guattari to Patrice Chéreau and Daniel Guérin, member of the Front homosexuel d'action révolutionnaire (Homosexual Front of Revolutionary Action), signed an opinion piece published in *Le Monde*[19] and *Libération* in defence of three men imprisoned for sexually abusing minors under the age of 15.

On 23 May 1977, 80 French intellectuals, including Michel Foucault, Roland Barthes, Alain Robbe-Grillet, Jacques Derrida, Philippe Sollers and Françoise Dolto, signed an open letter to the Commission de Revision du Code Pénal (Commission for the Revision of the Penal Code) asking it to decriminalise sexual relations between adults and children under the age of 15. Their demands were temporarily thwarted by the feminist movements and by the worldwide repercussions of the Dutroux affair[20].

Even so, the last ten years or so have seen the sexualisation of children gather pace with the perverse insistence on "learning" sexual gestures at school[21] along with the existence of rooms for exploring nudity and sexual games in day nurseries in Germany. Sexual practices have been compulsorily taught to German children since around 2014, and recalcitrant parents risk imprisonment[22] if

19. https://www.lemonde.fr/archives/article/1977/01/26/a-propos-d-un-proces_2854399_1819218.html

20. Major paedophile case that shook Belgium to its core.

21. https://www.lepoint.fr/monde/allemagne-preservatifs-positions-et-plaisir-au-menu-des-cours-d-education-sexuelle-15-02-2015-1905241_24.php

22. German parents in prison: testimony from Mathias Ebert, founder of "Besorgte Eltern" https://www.objectiondelaconscience.org/allemagne-des-parents-en-prison-parce-que-leur-enfant-ne-souhaitait-pas-assister-cours-deduction-sexuelle-en-primaire/

they refuse to allow their child to attend these very special sessions.

**Gender theorist Christopher Dummitt[23] and his confession**

Normal people wonder how such an ideology, which from its outset has denied the two-sex foundations of humanity, has been able to proliferate so widely in society, independently of the financial and social interests[24] that have been its secondary (often major) benefits.

One of the answers may lie in the enthusiasm of a certain number of academics who are jaded by their subject matter, bored to death and keen therefore to come up with "new" ideas that will relegate all the older generations to a bygone era. How easy it is for a teenager to call his father a "has-been" and close himself off to any discussion, after exposure to a few videos by influencers or to academics whose voices have reach ? Christopher Dummitt's statements[25] are a highly instructive case in point.

---

23. *Le Point*, "Canadian historian and expert in gender studies admits to falsifying his research findings in the service of his own political ideology" (04/11/2019).

24. If you're hoping to get a job in academia, you have to choose the subjects that are fashionable, in vogue, set by the agenda of the current power players. In medicine, since the '70s and '80s, it's been genetics, genetics, everything-genetics. All budgets went to laboratories submitting research projects on genetics and its many derivatives. In other fields, crumbs at best. But money is the lifeblood of any research project, whether it's hiring researchers, buying equipment, or whatever. In sociology, it was clearly feminist and then gender issues that filled the faculties and the posts of professors, lecturers, teaching fellows and so on.

25. Christopher Dummitt, a Canadian cultural and political historian, teaches at Trent University in Canada. He is the author of Unbuttoned : A History of Mackenzie King's Secret Life and of leading academic works on gender studies. According to his theory, sex is not a biological reality but a social construct, and gender, whether masculine or feminine, is a question of power, affirming the domination of men over women.

> "If I had known, 20 years ago, that my side in the ideological wars over gender and sex was going to win so decisively, I would have been ecstatic [...] I insisted that there was no such thing as sex. And I knew it, I just knew it. Because I was a gender historian".

This was, in the 1990s, the thing to be in history departments across North America. Gender history – and then gender studies, more generally, across the academy – was part of a broader group of identity-based sub-disciplines that were taking over the liberal arts. When the American Historical Association surveyed the trends among major fields of specialization in 2007, and then again in 2015, the single largest field was women's and gender history, followed closely by social history, cultural history, and the history of race and sexuality.
Christopher Dummitt was astonished at the speed at which academic thought has evolved, becoming a "pensée unique" in the space of thirty years:

> "If you take the position that many of my '90s-era debating opponents took—that gender is at least partly based on sex, and that there really are two sexes (male and female), as biologists have known since the dawn of their science – uber-progressives will claim you are denying a trans person's identity, which is to say, wishing ontological harm upon another human being. That's what makes it so amazing that the cultural turnaround on this issue has happened so quickly."

He admits to the falsification of his publications in the interests of his ideology.

> What I can offer is a mea culpa [...]. I also published an article out of my Master's thesis, which probably had a wider reach than my scholarly work. This was a fun article called Finding a Place for Father: Selling the Barbecue [26], which looked at the connection between men and barbecuing in Canada in the 1940s and 1950s. (Yes, this is the sort of thing that academics do.) First published back in 1998, it has been republished several times in textbooks for undergraduate students. […] I basically just made it up. In my defence, I wasn't alone. Everyone was (and is) making it up. That's how the gender-studies field works. But it's not much of a defence. I should have known better. My research didn't prove anything either way. I just assumed that gender was a social construct and proceeded on that basis".

He points out that the worst thing is that no one, especially his peers who should have critically re-read his articles, asked him to explain his results, but instead asked him "*to strengthen the paradigm, or to fight for other identities and rail against other forms of oppression*"[27].
In short, no one wanted him to justify what he was saying, nor did they criticise *the "extrapolation of his results"* for ideological purposes. On the contrary, all that was sought was use of his dominant academic position to extend this delusional theory even further.

---

26. This is curiously reminiscent of recent statements by French ecologists such as Sandrine Rousseau in 2023.
27. Peer review is nothing more than "the ideological scrutiny of an insider group", a tendency that has been observed in all areas of science over the last twenty years or so, leading to the serious consequences with which we are all familiar, including the marketing of dangerous experimental mRNA substances.

It is sad to note that this brave and instructive *mea culpa*, published in 2019 in Australia (the magazine *Quillette*[28]), and quoted in France (Atlantico[29] and *Le Point*[30] websites), and in Canada (on nouveau-monde.ca), was completely ignored by the Western media. Gender propaganda continued as if nothing had happened, the opinion of an academic specialist being of interest only if it aligns with the lobbies.

> "My flawed reasoning, and other scholarship using the same defective thinking, now is being taken up by activists and governments to legislate a new moral code of conduct [...]."

**What then, in 2023, do we call gender dysphoria?**[31]

According to Pauline Quillon, "dysphoria" means distress, unease or, more simply, discomfort. "Gender dysphoria" refers to a psychological state of discomfort, even malaise, in relation to the sex assigned at birth. So why use the word "gender" rather than "sex"? The word gender allows us to *distance* ourselves from material reality, and to introduce the idea that there may be a conflict between physiological sex and experienced sex; for example, a little girl may feel more like a boy than a girl.

---

28. https://quillette.com/2019/09/17/i-basically-just-made-it-up-confessions-of-a-social-constructionist/
29. https://atlantico.fr/article/pepite/christopher-dummitt-un-historien-canadien-fait-son-mea-culpa-sur-la-question-des-gender-studies-et-sur-ses-travaux
30. https://www.lepoint.fr/debats/theorie-du-genre-confessions-d-un-homme-dangereux-03-11-2019-2344979_2.php
31. Pauline Quillon, *Enquête sur la dysphorie de genre. Bien comprendre pour aider vraiment les enfants*, Mame, March 2022.

> "This psychological quirk has always existed. What's new is that this malaise has become dogma, denying the intangible, objective reality of sex and establishing its pseudo-fluidity from one extreme to the other".

## When social engineering turns the Western world into an open-air psychiatric hospital

Pauline Quillon's book shows how "philosophers" such as Judith Butler have exploited this eternal problem for ideological and political ends, using manipulation to stir up trouble among parents who are well-intentioned but ill-equipped to resist the social engineering set in motion, transforming more or less balanced societies into open-air psychiatric hospitals.

Some of the medical professions have themselves been won over by these innovative concepts, allowing them to dream of innovation and dispel their dreary ideas of everyday life. Some of them have also opened up highly lucrative markets and, like sociologists, obtained professorships and departments created to this end.

> "The child is then subjected to a terrible process, where drugs and surgery are combined, each fraught with adverse effects, creating irreversible physiological and psychological changes, without ever achieving the desired sex change. At the end of these manipulations, the boy or girl has become a new being, a "trans" person."

But what happens to these new transformed "Humans", the blueprint for augmented beings, the dream of some transhumanists? They take refuge in LGBTQ+ groups (and others with variations similar to this acronym), which are exerting an ever-greater philosophical, sociological and therefore political influence in most Western countries, transforming the democracy of the majority into a veritable tyranny of the minority. The individual meanwhile remains alone, isolated, unhappy, depressed and, before long, suicidal.

## Gender theory propaganda

Over the last thirty years or so, gender theory has permeated the content of TV series and films, particularly those on Netflix or Disney, in which minorities must tokenistically feature : a disabled person, a person of African origin, a male and/or female homosexual couple, if possible a transgender person, endeavouring not to overlook any minority (except Asians, who are most often ignored).

Political discourse has to be benevolent towards these active minorities for it to be considered right-thinking, on the side of good and therefore presentable in the media. Public media broadcasters that claim to be neutral, such as France Info, France Culture, France Inter and others, carefully weed out anyone who is not politically correct, thereby impoverishing their content and limiting proper democratic debate. Those who resist this ideology of feelings, such as Georgia Meloni (and even Elisabeth Badinter, wife of the minister responsible for President Mitterrand's abolition of the death penalty in France) are labelled reactionaries, homophobes, extreme right-wingers, fascists or post-fascists, or even anti-Semites.

## Trans identity propaganda specifically targets young people

"*Are you a child suffering from gender dysphoria who needs chemicals to block puberty*? According to London's Tavistock Gender Identity Clinic, most children need them. The clinic operated with impunity for forty years until it was closed by the NHS[32] after investigations found that the Tavistock was diagnosing and treating gender dysphoria in children, even if they were not suffering from it.

With transsexuality being widely promoted as a concept by the corporate media, leftist parents, state school teachers and many Western governments, it is no wonder that so many children are beginning to feel the need to jump on the bandwagon and signal their allegiance to the side of good. By and large, children want to make the adults around them happy, and the pressure to conform to sexual identity trends is immense. Tavistock, Britain's only sex and gender reassignment clinic in Britain, went from around 130 child patients a year in 2010 to almost 2,400 by 2021.

## Differences with the feminism of the past

As the feminism of the 80s waned, neo-feminists used the by-products of gender theory to fuel their discourse at a time when obtaining contraception, the extended right to abortion[33], and the expansion of women's place in politics and business were stifling some of their de-

32. National Health Service, Britain's equivalent to France's Ministère de la Santé.

33. Including in the ninth month of pregnancy.

mands. This weaponisation of feminist movements by transgender people led to their break-up, resulting in the realisation by a large proportion of historical feminists that the demands of trans women were detrimental to the recognition of womanhood, depriving them of the sporting titles they deserve (inclusivity of trans women in top-level women's sport) and threatening their safety (in prisons, changing rooms, dormitories, toilets).

**Even Family Planning is helping to erase women through language**

In the Family Planning lexicon, we can read that "*sex is a social construct*", that "*sex is a spectrum*", that a gay man "*can have a vulva*", that a lesbian couple can be made up of a woman and a trans woman (i.e. a male). Family Planning also encourages people to stop using the words "male" and "female". In short, within Family Planning, feminism is dead, since the very concept of "woman" has disappeared.

We have noticed that Family Planning now uses terms like "*menstruating person*", or "*people who have a womb*" to define women. "*We are opposed to this semantic division of women. We want to be seen as whole beings and not as vaginas on legs.*"[34]

34. « Mme Élisabeth Borne, féministes, nous nous inquiétons de ce que devient le Planning familial. » (marianne.net)

# 2.
# The consequences of medical treatment for gender dysphoria

Taking medication for the rest of your life when you are in good health is an aberration, madness even, given just the medical and physiological repercussions on the body at any age, but particularly when young.

The decision to prescribe hormones for gender reassignment is particularly complex, both medically and ethically. The medical treatments used for medical gender transition, such as luteinising hormone-releasing hormones[35] and/or so-called gender-affirming hormones[36], have major implications for growth, bone density, cardiovascular health and fertility. Their complications over a few months or years are known, but their long-term impact is unknown or poorly understood, due to the lack of hindsight and the absence of follow-up for the oldest patient cohorts.

35. LHRH.

36. Oestrogen for feminisation, or testosterone for masculinisation.

**“Changing gender” means a lifetime of major treatments**

This surely is the first piece of information that young people should be given before they embark on an experience that will all too often be tragic for them, in the longer or shorter term. After all, you can change the way you look, but not your biological sex or chromosomes. Changing your gender means deceiving your body (and others) for the rest of your life. And at what cost? That is what we will set out to explain as factually as possible, without making any value judgements. As doctors, when we use dangerous drugs to treat life-threatening illnesses such as cancer, we must assess the risk-benefit ratio and inform patients accordingly.

Our absolute rule of “first do no harm” applies all the more here because candidates for sex reassignment are not ill when they seek to initiate a “transition”. By trying to be of service to them and meet their demands, we run the risk of making them sick for life. This may be their adult choice, which we respect and will respect, but they must be fully informed.

In our opinion as paediatricians, hormone treatments and puberty blockers for transgender [37] [38] [39] purpos-

37. Kulesa R., “Toward a Standard of Medical Care: Why Medical Professionals Can Refuse to Prescribe Puberty Blockers.” *New Bioeth.* 2023 Jun.; 29(2):139-155. doi: 10.1080/20502877.2022.2137906. Epub 2022 Oct. 31. PMID: 36315442.

38. Giordano S., Garland F., Holm S. “Gender dysphoria in adolescents: can adolescents or parents give valid consent to puberty blockers?” *J Med Ethics.* 2021 Mar. 10: medethics-2020-106999. doi: 10.1136/medethics-2020-106999. Epub ahead of print. PMID: 33692171.

39. Known as gender dysphoria: causing unease in one’s body because it does not match their sense of identity.

es should be banned, especially in children, teenagers and young adults, whose bodies are not yet fully mature and will not be until they are over 25 (as the brain in particular is maturing). The real and potentially serious dangers of hormonal drugs are all too often underestimated not only by those applying to transition, but also by prescribers, who play down the effects to their "clients". The latter should be warned not only of the minor inconveniences that occur in the first few months, but above all of the potential medium- and long-term complications of these substances.

Puberty blockers are medicines that inhibit the production of sex hormones, thereby suspending puberty in the children and adolescents who receive them. They prevent adolescents from acquiring secondary sexual characteristics (voice changes, body transformations, breasts, pubic hair, beard according to their biological sex, penis size). The combination of puberty blockers and hormones to develop the appearance of the other sex will have irreversible consequences, even if they are discontinued. Several studies show that these puberty blockers do not reduce the risk of suicide[40].

These blockers also block other phenomena linked to puberty, such as growth, libido, bone calcification and fertility. These "gender-affirming"[41] hormone therapies

40. Dyer C. "Puberty blockers do not alleviate negative thoughts in children with gender dysphoria, finds study." *BMJ.* 2021 Feb. 8; 372: n356. doi: 10.1136/bmj.n356. PMID: 33558256.

41. According to the term used by doctors in this speciality. A misleading term, because the patient will only be able to "affirm" their choice without actually changing sex, only their physical appearance.

can lead to hypofertility and/or infertility[42]. If hormone therapy is used early in the puberty process, one of its effects is to render the person sterile by preventing the gametes from reaching full maturity. It should never be prescribed without rigorous medical supervision and clear information to allow truly informed consent[43], and never by self-prescribing via the Internet (all too easy to find through the good graces of network forums).

**Why are these hormones usually used outside of gender transitions?**

The treatment for early puberty, a real disease that affects a few children each year[44], is based essentially on the use of GnRH agonists[45], a hormonal medication. Slow-re-

42. Krebs D., Harris R. M., Steinbaum A., Pilcher S., Guss C., Kremen J., Roberts S. A., Baskaran C., Carswell J., Millington K. "Care for Transgender Young People." *Horm Res Paediatr.* 2022; 95(5):405-414. doi: 10.1159/000524030. Epub 2022 Mar. 10. PMID: 35272283; PMCID: PMC9463393.

43. Latham A. "Puberty Blockers for Children: Can They Consent?" *New Bioeth.* 2022 Sep.; 28(3):268-291. doi: 10.1080/20502877.2022.2088048. Epub 2022 Jun. 27. PMID: 35758886.

44. A child who develops, for example, at the age of 5 all the secondary sexual characteristics that normally appear from the age of 11-12: breasts, pubic hair, menstruation, etc.

45. From puberty to the menopause, oestrogens are mainly produced naturally by the ovaries, through a cascade process. The first component of this cascade is LHRH, a hormone produced by the hypothalamus. LHRH stimulates the pituitary gland (located at the base of the brain), which in response secretes a hormone, LH (luteinizing hormone), which in turn stimulates the ovaries to secrete oestrogen.

An agonist (or analogue) is a substance that resembles another substance and can therefore take its place and play its role by posing as it. The administration of LHRH analogues results in hyperstimulation of the pituitary gland. Once hyperstimulated, the pituitary gland will eventually stop responding and in turn stop stimulating the ovaries. Oestrogen production is thus halted. These drugs, used to block the actual disorder (precocious pulease, monthly or quarterly injections are used. These drugs effectively block and delay the process of puberty in an attempt to start it at the regular average age.

These are the same drugs that are used on children who are not ill, but who have announced that they feel they are a different sex. The major issue is the policy of affirmation[46] in this area on the part of doctors, some of whom are taking advantage of the situation to sell their business while others are proselytising their ideology.

As things stand in France, if a child, even a young one, claims to be of another sex, following the consent of the legal guardian[47], all medical, welfare, school and family professionals must abide by this decision, with no further discussion, nor even psychological counselling at present. The dangers of self-medication are well known and denounced by everyone, including the Académie de Médecine[48]. In no illness does the patient decide on the diagnosis, or indeed the treatment, which must be explained by the doctor to the patient in an effort to persuade them to accept it if deemed necessary. It must never be the patient who prescribes unilaterally and independently of the opinion of all the others. Moreover, people undergoing sex reassignment surgery are no longer considered to be "patients" (although curiously all treatment is ful-

---

berty) in certain children, are also used in other diseases to block hormone secretion, for example in patients with breast or prostate cancer. LH-RH agonists - Hormone therapy (e-cancer.fr)

46. According to trans activists, the fact of feeling trans is proof enough and justifies taking medical treatment without the need for a medical consultation.

47. https://www.gouvernement.fr/sites/default/files/contenu/piece jointe/2019/11/fiche_respect_des_droits_trans_dilcrah.pdfx

48. https://www.academie-medecine.fr/de-lautodiagnostic-a-lautomedication-risques-et-impact-sur-la-relation-pharmacien-patient/

ly reimbursed) yet are turned into actual patients by the medical treatments prescribed.

Children should have even less say in their own treatment! Imagine a child with a bone tumour who wants to choose which chemotherapy regimen to use or refuses it simply on the basis of their feelings. Parents who accept the dictates of their sick offspring who refuse treatment would be sent before a children's court judge and their guardianship would be withdrawn. A child is not responsible before the law (by reason of minority status), cannot vote in elections, nor drive a car… And yet, to facilitate gender reassignment, the lobbies have imposed their fantasies (as they themselves describe them) and minors have every right, regardless of the wishes of their parents, or in some countries without their knowledge. To say otherwise is to be declared transphobic and liable to prosecution.

Abroad, where these practices have been widespread for a long time, the number of lawsuits brought against carers who have driven minors too quickly into this transition is multiplying. The number of such cases and the problems they highlight have led many health authorities to ban gender reassignment treatments for minors or to restrict them to official clinical trials[49 50]. We shall return to this point later.

49. Mahase E. "Puberty blockers for young people will only be available as part of clinical research", says NHS England. *BMJ*. 2023 Jun. 12; 381: 1344. doi: 10.1136/bmj.p1344. PMID: 37308216.

50. Dyer C. "Puberty blockers: children under 16 should not be referred without court order", says NHS England. *BMJ*. 2020 Dec. 2; 371: m4717. doi: 10.1136/bmj.m4717. PMID: 33268453.

Developed in the 1980s to treat precocious puberty, drugs based on male or female hormones have transformed the treatment of transgender people ever since they were first used for this purpose in the late 1990s, giving rise to the dire consequences that were denied at the time and are still downplayed too often in the media in 2023.
The Endocrine Society explicitly recommends that puberty should not be blocked before its onset[51]. A doctor who administers blockers to a 5-6-year-old child in the wrong way is halting the development of puberty[52], which may never take place normally.
A child, on reaching the age for natural puberty, will receive a cross-over hormone treatment if he or she still wants to transition (often surrounded by militant doctors and carers who, for ideological reasons, entertain no doubts). If a girl wants to become a man, she will receive male hormones - testosterone - and conversely a boy who wants to become a girl will receive female hormones, i.e. oestrogen. These are the hormones that older adults wishing to change sex will also receive.

## Becoming feminised

The treatment is carried out with natural oestrogens, through the skin, or with natural progesterone and finasteride (in the case of hair loss). Feminising hormone

51. Gender Dysphoria/Gender Incongruence Guideline Resources. https://www.endocrine.org/clinical-practice-guidelines/gender-dysphoria-gender-incongruence
52. Kulesa R. "Toward a Standard of Medical Care: Why Medical Professionals Can Refuse to Prescribe Puberty Blockers." New Bioeth. 2023 Jun.; 29(2):139-155. doi: 10.1080/20502877.2022.2137906. Epub 2022 Oct. 31. PMID: 36315442.

treatment[53] has reversible effects, but also certain irreversible consequences. Even if one's character does not always change, which is not obvious given the devastating effects on morale and depression, the usual reversible effects are a reduction in musculature, a change in the distribution of fat, reduced sweating, and a decrease in blood pressure, red blood cells and body heat. Certain irreversible effects need to be taken into account : the breasts develop significantly ; the areolas widen and stretch marks appear. In transgender women (born male), a combination of testosterone blockers[54] and oestrogen treatment is necessary. Testosterone inhibitors are necessary because testosterone acts more strongly in the body than oestrogen. But there are many negative effects : reduced libido, changes in cholesterol and cardiovascular effects, and others[55]. Bicalutamide, an androgen receptor blocker, has been associated with fulminant liver failure in prostate cancer treatment[56]. Endocrinology Society guidelines[57] specifically suggest that oral ethinylestradiol should not be used in transgender women, as it is very frequently associat-

53. Les traitements hormonaux féminisants – Vivre Trans (vivre-trans.fr)
54. Via spironolactone or removal of the testicles = orchiectomy.
55. A number of physiological markers that affect cardiovascular health. C-reactive protein, insulin-like growth factor, angiotensin (a protein in the blood), other liver proteins. These changes can lead to increased blood clotting and reduced cardiovascular health. They are not often seen, if at all, with non-oral oestrogens.
56. Hussain S., Haidar A., Bloom R. E., Zayouna N., Piper M. H., Jafri S. M. R. Bicalutamide-induced hepatotoxicity : A rare adverse effect The American Journal of Case Reports, 2014 ; 15 : 266–70. 10.12659/AJCR.890679. https://www.ncbi.nlm.nih.gov/pmc/articles/PMC9463393/
57. Wylie C. Hembree et al. Endocrine Treatment of Gender-Dysphoric/Gender-Incongruent Persons : An Endocrine Society Clinical Practice Guideline Downloaded from https://academic.oup.com/jcem/article/102/11/3869/4157558 by Withers user on 24 August 2023.

ed with thromboembolic events (deep vein thrombosis, heart attack, pulmonary embolism and stroke).
All the studies confirm that the risk of developing venous thromboembolism, i.e. the formation of a blood clot, is clearly higher in transgender women than in non-transgender men (risk multiplied by 5 after two years' follow-up) and native-born women (risk multiplied by 3). As for the risk of stroke caused by a blood clot, the probabilities were 9.9 times higher in transgender women than in men in the control group and 4.1 times higher than in women in the control group, after a follow-up period of more than six years in the cited study[58].

**Becoming masculinised**
In transgender men, testosterone can lead to acne, baldness, weight gain, increased red blood cell count, increased cholesterol and elevated liver enzymes. It can also contribute to the development of hypertension, type 2 diabetes and cardiovascular disease.

**Lifelong patient**
Whichever oestrogen treatments, or conversely masculinising hormones, are used, medical supervision is important. The doctor must monitor hormone levels in the blood. These high-risk drugs require lifelong monitoring for all transgender people undergoing treatment.
Is this the paradise on Earth that the dream merchants, and most importantly the purveyors of repeated medication and surgery, have led them to imagine? Parents

58. Changement de sexe : prendre des hormones n'est pas sans risque pour la santé cardiovasculaire (pourquoidocteur.fr)

should think very carefully before involving their child in such a medical experiment. Is becoming a lifelong patient an option ? Ask those who made no such choice and who are suffering from congenital disease, cancer, chronic illnesses, neurological disorders, and so forth, what they would have done had they been given the choice.

Isn't the first vow and commitment in our Hippocratic oath *primum non nocere* ("above all, do no harm") ? First imperative : clear communication to patients.

**Transgender people : twice the mortality risk**[59]
Transgender people are twice as likely to die as cisgender people. The causes vary according to gender.
Suicide : one of the leading causes of death in transgender men.
An observational study published in the journal *The Lancet Diabetes & Endocrinology* by Amsterdam doctors promoting transsexual treatments found an increased risk of mortality among transgender people using hormonal treatment, regardless of treatment type. In transgender women, the risk of mortality was almost twice as high compared with cisgender men and almost three times as high compared with cisgender women. In naturally born women who became transgender men, the risk was similar to that of cisgender men, but almost double that of cisgender women. This increased risk of mortality did not decrease over the five decades of

59. "Mortality trends over five decades in adult transgender people receiving hormone treatment : a report from the Amsterdam cohort of gender dysphoria" – *The Lancet Diabetes & Endocrinology.*

the study (1978 to 2018), which belies, among other things, previous claims that treatments reduce the risk of suicide. This article attempts to exonerate the role of drugs in this excess mortality, but nevertheless acknowledges that the data are insufficient. It is comparable to the mystification at work in denying the role of anti-Covid gene therapy in the current epidemic of sudden deaths.

Young people are all too often told that gender transition procedures are completely reversible and well-managed, or that people who regret their decision are extremely rare (which is not true, as we shall come back to), but one of the causes of these underestimates is the lack of frequent follow-up for those who have undergone the operation.

The glamour and glitter of Angela Ponce (who represented Spain at the Miss Universe 2018 pageant in Bangkok), who says she "*wants to be a role model for transgender children*", overshadows the many very real drawbacks associated with gender transition.

In 2015, four US gender transition clinics received $7 million to examine the effects of hormone blockers and treatments on young transgender people. In justifying their funding request, the researchers pointed out that the US had produced no data on the impact or safety of blockers, particularly in transgender patients under the age of 12, leaving a "*gap in the evidence base for this practice*". By 2022, they had yet to report the main findings of their work, but claimed that the results would be available soon. In 2023, we are still waiting for them.

## Analysis of the impact of hormone therapy when initiated during adolescence

A survey carried out in Portugal among transgender people who were undergoing or had undergone hormone therapy for at least one uninterrupted year revealed that 89 % of them had experienced side-effects. Across all genders, more than half complained of emotional problems and 10 % experienced recurrent headaches. In addition, 66 % of men undergoing feminisation reported a loss of libido. Among women who are becoming masculinised, 52.9 % suffer from acne, 38 % from hair loss and 25 % from pelvic pain. As for men undergoing feminisation, 15 % experience nausea and 15 % suffer from itching associated with exanthema.

## Cardiovascular risk of hormone therapy

In both groups, the incidence of cardiovascular problems was higher than in the general population[60] despite the usual preventive measures (smoking cessation, dietary care, combating sedentary behaviour), which are essential in this particularly vulnerable population[61].

---

60. Santos R. B., Lemos C., Saraiva M., "Gender-Affirming Hormone Therapy: Physical and Sociopsychological Effects, Impact and Satisfaction." *Cureus*. 2023 Mar. 21 ; 15(3).
61. Nicolaï Johnson, Nathalie Chabbert-Buffet, « Hormonothérapie féminisante chez les femmes transgenres », *La Presse Médicale Formation*, Vol. 1, No. 6, December 2020, pages 597-603.

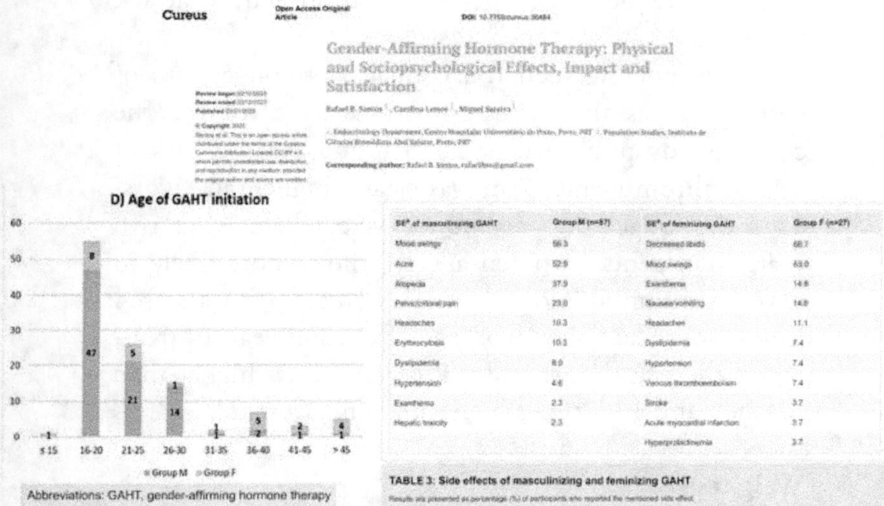


| SE* of masculinizing GAHT | Group M (n=87) | SE* of feminizing GAHT | Group F (n=27) |
|---|---|---|---|
| Mood swings | 56.3 | Decreased libido | 66.7 |
| Acne | 52.9 | Mood swings | 63.0 |
| Alopecia | 37.9 | Exanthema | 14.8 |
| Pelvic/clitoral pain | 23.0 | Nausea/vomiting | 14.8 |
| Headaches | 10.3 | Headaches | 11.1 |
| Erythrocytosis | 10.3 | Dyslipidemia | 7.4 |
| Dyslipidemia | 8.0 | Hypertension | 7.4 |
| Hypertension | 4.6 | Venous thromboembolism | 7.4 |
| Exanthema | 2.3 | Stroke | 3.7 |
| Hepatic toxicity | 2.3 | Acute myocardial infarction | 3.7 |
| | | Hyperprolactinemia | 3.7 |

TABLE 3: Side effects of masculinizing and feminizing GAHT

Results are presented as percentage (%) of participants who reported the mentioned side effect.

According to Dr Michael Irwing, Associate Professor at Harvard Medical School and Director for Transgender Medicine at Beth Israel in Boston, hormone therapies affect blood pressure. While hormone therapies lower blood pressure in men undergoing feminisation, they considerably increase it in transgender men (born female) who take testosterone : an average of 2.6 mm Hg, a not inconsiderable figure over a lifetime. The study of 470 patients[62] confirms the relatively high cardiovascular risk associated with hormone treatments, and after it was presented to the American Heart Association's cardiologists, the Association strongly recommended regular cardiological monitoring of transgender people

62. *Gender-Affirming Hormone Therapy May Increase Risk of Blood Pressure*, BIDMC of Boston.
"Cross-sex Hormones and Acute Cardiovascular Events in Transgender Persons : A Cohort Study" – *PubMed* (nih.gov).

on hormone therapies for early detection of heart attack and stroke.

In transgender women (born male), prolonged use of oestrogens has an impact on venous circulation[63]. The cohort study published in 2018 found that the risk of venous thromboembolism was clearly higher, and worsened the longer that hormones were taken. After two years, transgender women are 4.1 times more likely to develop thrombosis or a blood clot than men and 3.4 times more likely than women. After eight years of treatment, the risk rises sharply: it is 16.7 times higher than for men and 13.7 times higher than for women.

**Weight gain**

The results of a **longitudinal study**[64] in gender-affirming people show that their hormone treatment often leads to weight gain, particularly in women who transition to male.

The study reports that: in the 2 to 4 months following the start of hormone therapy, the average body weight had increased in the transgender male group (female to male) by 2.35 (1.15-3.55) kg and continued to increase beyond 34 months. In the transgender female group (male to female),

63. Asscheman H., T'Sjoen G., Lemaire A., Mas M., Meriggiola M. C., Mueller A., Kuhn A., Dhejne C., Morel-Journel N., Gooren L. J. "Venous thrombo-embolism as a complication of cross-sex hormone treatment of male-to-female transsexual subjects: a review." Andrologia. 2014 Sep.; 46(7):791-5. doi: 10.1111/and.12150. Epub 2013 Aug. 15. PMID: 23944849.

64. Kyinn, M., Banks, K., Leemaqz, S. Y. *et al.* "Weight gain and obesity rates in transgender and gender-diverse adults before and during hormone therapy." *Int J Obes* 45, 2562-2569 (2021). https://doi.org/10.1038/s41366-021-00935-x

mean body weight remained stable during the first 21 months of hormone therapy, then began to increase steadily, particularly in the under-30s. With a baseline prevalence of obesity of 25 % in the transgender female group and 39 % in the transgender male group, obesity rates rose from 42 % to 52 % in the transgender male group and from 21 % to 30 % in the transgender female group.
After 11 to 21 months of hormone therapy, weight gain ≥5 kg was observed in 21 % of transgender females and 30 % of transgender males.

**Reduced bone mass**

Feminising hormone therapy (oestrogens) significantly reduces bone mass, particularly in the lumbar spine[65] [66] [67], which could lead to an increased risk of fractures in transgender women.
A Swedish television documentary[68] reported the case of a transgender teenager who took these drugs between

65. Schagen S., Wouters F. M., Cohen-Kettenis P. T. , Gooren L. J., Hannema S. E. "Bone Development in Transgender Adolescents Treated With GnRH Analogues and Subsequent Gender-Affirming Hormones." J Clin Endocrinol Metab. 2020 Dec. 1 ; 105(12):e4252–63. doi : 10.1210/clinem/dgaa604. PMID : 32909025 ; PMCID : PMC7524308.
66. Lapauw B., Taes Y., Simoens S., Van Caenegem E., Weyers S., Goemaere S., Toye K., Kaufman J. M., T'Sjoen G. G. "Body composition, volumetric and areal bone parameters in male-to-female transsexual persons." Bone. 2008 Dec. ; 43(6):1016-21. doi : 10.1016/j.bone.2008.09.001. Epub 2008 Sep. 16. PMID : 18835591.
67. Fighera T. M., Ziegelmann P. K., Rasia da Silva T., Spritzer P. M. "Bone Mass Effects of Cross-Sex Hormone Therapy in Transgender People" : Updated Systematic Review and Meta-Analysis. J Endocr Soc. 2019 Mar. 15 ; 3(5):943-964. doi : 10.1210/js.2018-00413. PMID : 31020058 ; PMCID : PMC6469959.
68. https://www.svtplay.se/video/33358590/uppdrag-granskning/mission-investigate-trans-children-avsnitt-1?info=visa

the ages of 11 and 14 and developed osteoporosis with a compression fracture of the spine. "*The patient now suffers from continued back pain*", the medical records note, describing a "*permanent disability*" caused by puberty blockers.

**Puberty blockers also have an as yet poorly understood impact on the brain**

Some doctors and researchers fear that puberty blockers could in some way disrupt this formative period of mental growth. Adolescence is accompanied by critical thinking, more sophisticated personal reflection and other significant advances in brain development.

Sex hormones have been shown to affect social and problem-solving skills. Brain growth is thought to be linked to gender, but research in these areas is still very new. In Finland, doctors remain concerned about the physical effects of blockers, particularly on brain development, said Dr Riittakerttu Kaltiala, head of adolescent psychiatry at a gender clinic in Tampere.

**Permanent infertility** is likely for those who have taken the drugs from an early age - a crucial decision for children who cannot grasp the far-reaching implications of these decisions. Our bodies are programmed from conception. Male and female organisms are programmed to produce, manage and convert hormones in different ways. For example, a certain amount of enzyme is needed to produce oestrogen or to eliminate the by-products of testosterone.

Men's oestrogen levels vary from around 0 to 40 picograms, whereas women's levels are 5 to 10 times higher.

Knowing that cytochromes P450[69] are involved in the metabolism of oestrogen, a transgender woman (born male) will be ill-equipped to deal with the sudden influx of this hormone, taken for many years as part of a gender affirmation process.
Moreover, hormones are in balance with each other and this can influence our general metabolism[70], with repercussions on other organs. Oestrogen therapy can inhibit the proper functioning of the liver by reducing hepatic lipase activity by up to 64 % and lipoprotein lipase activity by up to 23 %. This may, for example, increase the risk of kidney stones. These changes require constant clinical and biological monitoring to detect the complications inherent in these medical manipulations, which are by no means natural and are not without risks to individual health, as borne out by the increased all-cause mortality rates among transgender people at the Amsterdam clinic[71].
As with all treatments, particularly those that are extensive and prolonged, good medical practice requires that the person being considered for treatment undergo a thorough clinical and laboratory assessment at the outset. However, this is not always the case for candidates being considered for sex reassignment hormone therapy.

---

69. "Cytochrome P450-mediated metabolism of estrogens and its regulation in human" – *PubMed* (nih.gov)
70. "A review of the physical and metabolic effects of cross-sex hormonal therapy in the treatment of gender dysphoria" – Leighton J. Seal, 2016 (sagepub.com)
71. *Ibid.*, 51.

## The great hormonal disorder and endocrine disruptors

Those seeking transition may include not only healthy people choosing to change gender, but also people suffering from a little-known disease that might explain their malaise, such as perhaps a hormonal imbalance, leading them to think that they are in the wrong body. As a result of fashion trends, influencers and ideologues, these people are being steered far too quickly towards this assumption during medical consultations and/or on social media before seeking a clinical diagnosis to explain symptoms that could be treated simply. So many diseases go unnoticed because they are not investigated.

In an episode of *The Highwire*[72] on the safety of hormone therapy drugs, endocrinologist Dr Patrick Flynn reports a case where a young woman with acne problems and a lot of body hair broke down in tears when she confessed that she often felt "as if she were a man" and that she wondered about her gender identity. In addition to these rather masculine characteristics, she also reported excessive moodiness and aggressive behaviour. The doctor was quick to reassure her, explaining that hormonal imbalances can throw us off-kilter, and ordered extensive tests which revealed that her testosterone levels were far too high. Finally, once her endocrine function had returned to normal, the young woman's physical and mental health improved, and she proudly announced that she "felt good about her femininity again".

Unfortunately, endocrine disorders are on the increase due to a variety of environmental factors in particular,

72. "Are gender transition drugs safe ?" – *The HighWire.*

and should be investigated before all else in this "gender identity" saga. Journalist Corinne Lalo published *Le grand désordre hormonal*[73] and believes that we are currently facing a widespread hormonal imbalance, the cause of a deterioration in human and animal health.

> "Fish are becoming feminised, snails are seeing the appearance of females with penises, alligators now have micropenises, ibises are becoming homosexuals… In humans, boys have testicles that no longer descend, men are losing half their spermatozoa in one generation, and their testosterone levels are falling significantly… Girls are going through puberty early, young women are having painful periods, and breast cancer is on the increase in women."

Shouldn't we, therefore, first restore the hormonal health of the candidate for transition by investigating the possibility of an undiagnosed endocrine disorder, before taking the risk of aggravating it and concluding too quickly that they are "trans-identifying"? But for that to happen, we absolutely must put an end to the imbecilic and totalitarian rule of the subject affirming his or her identity, regardless of the opinion of his or her family, friends, medical environment, and so forth.

The sharp increase in the number of young people who feel uncomfortable in their skin and who may feel themselves to be of a different sex could be linked, in part, to the proliferation of endocrine disruptors from pesticides, plastics, and other materials that interfere with prenatal

73. Corinne Lalo, *Le Grand désordre hormonal. Ce qui nous empoisonne à notre insu*, Le Cherche-Midi, 2021.

and postnatal development - in short, all the components of our industrial diet.

A survey conducted by Dr Scott Kerlin among sons exposed to DES[74] administered to pregnant women to prevent nausea, showed that 30 % of them became transgender. Elsewhere, poultry farmers have given DES to young roosters to turn them into hens[75].
Atrazine, a common pesticide, turns male frogs into egg-laying females, as documented by Tyrone B. Hayes of U.C. Berkeley[76]. These changes seem to become hereditary. It is by no means simple, but there is value in asking about family history and carrying out tests before rushing to take pills that look harmless to the young person, but are not.

And, of course, in a normal medical world, an indispensable first step would be to determine the psychological stability of candidates for transition before any medical procedures. Another would be to restore as far as possible the mental health of children and young people, who, over and above possible hormonal imbalances, have so many reasons to be disturbed, particularly in the wake

74. Diethylstilbestrol, the first synthetic oestrogen widely prescribed between 1940 and 1970. https://www.orpha.net/consor/cgi-bin/OC_Exp.php?Expert=1916&lng=FR see also on FB "les filles du DES".
75. See Toxic Bodies, Langston, p. 66.
76. Hayes T. B. , Khoury V., Narayan A., Nazir M., Park A., Brown T., Adame L., Chan E., Buchholz D., Stueve T., Gallipeau S. "Atrazine induces complete feminization and chemical castration in male African clawed frogs (Xenopus laevis)." *Proc Natl Acad Sci USA*. 2010 Mar 9; 107(10):4612-7. doi: 10.1073/pnas.0909519107. Epub 2010 Mar 1. PMID: 20194757; PMCID: PMC2842049.

of the recent Covid pandemic, with its procession of delusional and contradictory measures leading to a state of general cognitive dissonance.
Statistics on depression and psychiatric disorders among young people show that the frequency of these disorders has exploded. Against this backdrop, how can we fail to demand psychological treatment before authorising these hormonal procedures, the lifelong consequences of which are known, even if they are discontinued[77] after a few years? The well-being of candidates for transition should be the primary concern of the doctors who treat them.

**The silence imposed on the medical consequences of hormones has resulted in too many tragedies**

Puberty blockers and cross hormones cause irreversible harm: can we finally talk about this without being prosecuted for transphobia?[78]
The puberty blockers officially prescribed to young people questioning their gender to "give them time to think" would only be conceivable if their effects were actually reversible and without harmful consequences. Unfortunately, this is not the case.
Until recently, books and articles denouncing the harmful consequences of these drugs were systematically vilified by transgender activists and censored in the media, as was the case with Abigail Shrier's *Irreversible Damage: The Transgender Craze Seducing Our Daughters*, a well-re-

77. On choosing to detransition, see the chapter dealing with this subject.
78. https://www.lifesitenews.com/blogs/even-the-new-york-times-is-worried-about-the-irreversible-damage-of-puberty-blockers

searched book named book of the year by *The Economist* and one of the best books of 2021 by *The Times*.
But with the growing number of children subjected to these treatments over a long period[79], the lies of the transgender lobbies, who constantly repeat that these drugs are harmless and their effects reversible, are becoming blatantly obvious.

The high suicide rate is one of the main features of transgender people's mental health compared with the general population. Several studies show that more than 40 % of transgender people have attempted suicide at least once in their lives[80] [81], almost 20 % more than heterosexuals and ten times more than homosexuals. Even the *New York Times* reports on the failures and complications of this hormone therapy for transsexuals in an article entitled "They Paused Puberty, But is There A Cost?"[82].
The sole merit of such admissions on the part of these transgender activists is that the tragic consequences of these treatments along with the mental derangement of our society are now in evidence. More and more transgender people are coming forward to tell their stories, one girl explaining, for example, that despite the sup-

79. In the United States, around 300,000 people aged between 13 and 17 and countless younger people identify themselves as transgender.
80. Chérie Moody et Nathan Grant Smith, "Suicide Protective Factors Among Trans Adults", *Archives of Sexual Behavior*, vol. 42, no 5, July 2013, p. 739-752.
81. Lore M. Dickey et Stephanie L. Budge, "Suicide and the transgender experience: A public health crisis.", *American Psychologist*, vol. 75, no 3, April 2020, p. 380-390.
82. Megan Twohey and Christina Jewett, "They Paused Puberty, but Is There a Cost?" *The New York Times*, November 14, 2022.

pression of male hormones, she has a permanently deep voice.

**What is the point of giving these treatments to children, 85 % of whom would have done without them had we taken the time to think and provide them with the necessary psychological support?**

> "About a dozen studies of gender-dysphoric children who did not take puberty blockers have found that most of them, if supported by counselling, are happy with their sex once they emerge from puberty. The share often cited is 85 % and many of them turn out to be gay.
> One sign that something is wrong is that more people are "de-transitioning"—re-identifying with their biological sex. Most of them are girls who wanted to be boys when they were in their teens. If they took puberty blockers and then cross-sex hormones early they would be sterile for life, even if they did not have hysterectomies"[83].

The trans "epidemic" that seems to be developing in our country (well after that of the Anglo-Saxon countries, which are seeing a decline) reflects a feeling of unease that is common in adolescence but is being used by the merchants of hope who are turning it into a very real business.
Even professionals and activists in the field of transitions acknowledge anomalies. According to the World Professional Association for Transgender Health (WPATH), gender reassignment surgery should only take place after

83. "What to do about puberty blockers", The Economist, 30 January 2020

an "*extensive exploration of psychological, family, and social issues*" is undertaken. This seems obvious.
All too often, however, gender dysphoria is not subject to medical examination. Existing research shows that most children who identify as belonging to the other sex eventually regain a sense of gender congruence on their own. They are also prone to depression and anxiety disorders. It is a complicated web to untangle for patients, their parents and health professionals, who have to determine which child in this group of cases is suffering from real gender dysphoria that will become permanent over time. Laura Edwards-Leeper, professor of psychology at Pacific University in Oregon and co-founder of the first clinic for transgender children in the United States, in Boston, admits that the "*vast majority of children on blockers or sex hormones have not undergone proper assessments*"[84]. If even they themselves are saying so…

**Sex reassignment treatments do not reduce the risk of suicide**

The main arguments used by pro-trans activists and associations to justify sex reassignment treatments are that they are not dangerous and that they reduce the risk of suicide, but they do not cite any long-term studies to back up their beliefs. However, doctors at the Amsterdam clinic, which was the first in Europe to administer these treatments, contradict these claims by reporting "*an increased mortality risk in transgender people using hormone treatment, regardless of treatment type. This in-*

84. *Ibid.*, 6.

*creased mortality risk did not decrease over time*"[85] (this risk is almost double that of the general population). They conclude their study of the risk of suicide over five decades as follows[86]: "*Suicide death risk in trans people did not increase over time. Suicide deaths occurred during every stage of transitioning.*"

IN FRANCE, VERY FEW PEOPLE SEEK SEX REASSIGNMENT SURGERY

Annual number of requests and approved payments by the Caisse National d'Assurance Maladie for sex reassignment surgery 2012-2020

| Year | Public Funding Requests for Breast and/or Pelvic Surgery | | total | % accepted |
|---|---|---|---|---|
| | Refused | Accepted | | |
| 2012 | 33 | 80 | 113 | 71% |
| 2013 | 59 | 106 | 165 | 64% |
| 2014 | 74 | 140 | 214 | 65% |
| 2015 | 61 | 146 | 207 | 71% |
| 2016 | 48 | 167 | 215 | 78% |
| 2017 | 88 | 187 | 275 | 68% |
| 2018 | 138 | 226 | 364 | 62% |
| 2019 | 170 | 320 | 490 | 65% |
| 2020 | 118 | 344 | 462 | 74% |

source CNAM

85. De Blok C. J. , Wiepjes C. M., van Velzen D. M., Staphorsius A. S., Nota N. M., Gooren L. J. , Kreukels B. P., den Heijer M. "Mortality trends over five decades in adult transgender people receiving hormone treatment: a report from the Amsterdam cohort of gender dysphoria." Lancet Diabetes Endocrinol. 2021 Oct.; 9(10):663-670. doi: 10.1016/S2213-8587(21)00185-6. Epub 2021 Sep. 2. PMID: 34481559.

86. Wiepjes C. M., den Heijer M., Bremmer M. A., Nota N. M., de Blok C. J. M., Coumou B. J. G., Steensma T. D. "Trends in suicide death risk in transgender people: results from the Amsterdam Cohort of Gender Dysphoria study (1972-2017)." Acta Psychiatr Scand. 2020 Jun.; 141(6):486-491. doi: 10.1111/acps.13164. Epub 2020 Mar. 12. PMID: 32072611; PMCID: PMC7317390.

# 3.
# Sex reassignment surgery: a long, difficult, irreversible and often unsatisfactory road

Sex reassignment surgery involves a series of procedures that change a person's physical appearance, so that it resembles the opposite sex as closely as possible.
Also known as "gender affirmation" or "gender confirmation" surgery, it is the irreversible stage of a transition process that gives, as closely as possible, to gender dysphoria sufferers the body they have been craving. Around one in four transgender people go on to have surgery.

In France, the number of transgender people undergoing surgery has quadrupled between 2012 and 2020, as shown in this table from the National Health Insurance Fund.

Gender transition normally begins with psychological preparation aimed at eliminating those suffering from psychosis or depression and attempting to explain to candidates for gender transition the irreversible consequences of the planned medical and surgical procedures[87]. This phase used to last two years but tends to be shorter nowadays under pressure from lobbies.

When the psychiatrist considers the patient ready and there are no contraindications (risk of cardiovascular accident, obesity, severe diabetes, hypertension, etc.), hormone therapy can begin, to which are added, more or less rapidly, surgical interventions. In France, transitions from male to female happen currently twice as often as the reverse.

**Possible procedures to transform a man into a trans woman**

These may involve operations on the face, glottis, chest[88] and/or genitals. Facial surgery[89 90] can involve modifying the appearance of the cheekbones using injections, of the

87. Dahlen S., Connolly D., Arif I., Junejo M. H., Bewley S., Meads C. "International clinical practice guidelines for gender minority/trans people: systematic review and quality assessment." BMJ Open. 2021 Apr. 29; 11(4):e048943. doi: 10.1136/bmjopen-2021-048943

88. Claes Key, d'Arpa S., Monstrey S. J. "Chest Surgery for Transgender and Gender Nonconforming Individuals." Clin Plast Surg. 2018 Jul; 45(3):369-380.

89. Hazkour N., Palacios J., Lu W., Goote P., Rivera R., Bastidas N. "Multiprocedural Facial Feminization Surgery: A Review of Complications in a Cohort of 31 Patients." *J Craniofac Surg.* 2022 Nov.-Dec. 01; 33(8):2502-2506. doi: 10.1097 Epub 2022 Jul. 26. PMID: 36102911.

90. Rodman R. "Developments in facial feminization surgery." *Curr Opin Otolaryngol Head Neck Surg.* 2022 Aug. 1; 30(4):249-253

chin to soften the angles, of the jaws to reduce the sharpness of the line, the nose to reshape it (rhinoplasty), the Adam's apple to make it invisible, not forgetting full and permanent hair removal.
Healing usually takes 2 to 4 weeks but it can take up to four months for any oedema to disappear after corrective surgery on the jaws. In the USA, full facial feminisation surgery can cost up to $52,500 [91].

**Glottoplasty**[92][93][94][95] and/or voice re-education are sometimes useful in order to avoid surprising interlocutors with tones that are too deep for the gender displayed[96][97].

---

91. https://www.gofundme.com/fr-fr/c/blog/gender-confirmation-surgery
92. Yılmaz T., Özer F., Aydınlı F. E. "Laser Reduction Glottoplasty for Voice Feminization: Experience on 28 Patients." *Ann Otol Rhinol Laryngol.* 2021 Sep.; 130(9):1057-1063. Epub 2021 Feb 10.
93. Husain S., Campe L., Mirza N. "Modification of Wendler Glottoplasty for Male to Female Gender Transition." *J Voice.* 2023 Mar. 24: S0892-1997(23)00027-9. doi: 10.1016/j.jvoice.2023.01.028. Epub ahead of print. PMID: 36967260.
94. Song T. E., Jiang N. "Transgender Phonosurgery: A Systematic Review and Meta-analysis." *Otolaryngol Head Neck Surg.* 2017 May; 156(5):803-808. doi: 10.1177/0194599817697050. Epub 2017 Mar. 28. PMID: 28349733.
95. McNeill EJ. "Management of the transgender voice." *J Laryngol Otol.* 2006 Jul.; 120(7):521-3.
96. Brown S. K., Chang J., Hu S., Sivakumar G., Sataluri M., Goldberg L., Courey M. S. "Addition of Wendler Glottoplasty to Voice Therapy Improves Trans Female Voice Outcomes." Laryngoscope. 2021 Jul.; 131(7):1588-1593. doi: 10.1002/lary.29050. Epub 2020 Aug 26.
97. Nolan I. T., Morrison S. D., Arowojolu O., Crowe C. S., Massie J. P., Adler R. K., Chaiet S. R., Francis D. O. "The Role of Voice Therapy and Phonosurgery in Transgender Vocal Feminization." *J Craniofac Surg.* 2019 Jul; 30(5):1368-1375.

**Breast augmentation** should wait until the size of the breasts has stabilised following hormonal therapy and is achieved by the insertion of implants[98], tissue expanders under the mammary gland or fat transplants from other parts of the body.

**Pelvic surgery** (feminising genitoplasty) involves the removal of the penis, testicles and scrotum and the construction of a vulva, usually followed by that of a vagina. It begins with the removal of the testicles and the penis.

**Vaginoplasty** is a complex surgery that lasts between 2 and 4 hours, often requires hospitalisation for 2 weeks[99][100] and results in complications in 70 % of cases[101][102]. Vaginoplasty by turning the penis inside out is the simplest of the techniques[103]; the skin of the "inverted" penis is

98. Post op Transgender Genitals, "What You Can Expect Post Op Bottom surgery?" | ClinicSpotshttps://www.clinicspots.com/blog/post-op-transgender-genitalia-surgery

99. https://sante.journaldesfemmes.fr/fiches-anatomie-et-examens/2554842-vaginoplastie-operation-transgenre/

100. Ferrando CA. "Updates on feminizing genital affirmation surgery (vaginoplasty) techniques." *Neurourol Urodyn.* 2023 Jun. ; 42(5):931-938. doi: 10.1002/nau.25088. Epub 2022 Nov. 24. PMID: 36423307.

101. Morrison S. D., Claes K., Morris M. P., Monstrey S., Hoebeke P., Buncamper M. "Principles and outcomes of gender-affirming vaginoplasty." *Nat Rev Urol.* 2023 May; 20(5):308-322. doi: 10.1038/s41585-022-00705-y. Epub 2023 Feb. 1. PMID: 36726039.

102. Jiang D., Witten J., Berli J., Dugi D 3rd. "Does Depth Matter? Factors Affecting Choice of Vulvoplasty Over Vaginoplasty as Gender-Affirming Genital Surgery for Transgender Women." *J Sex Med.* 2018 Jun. ; 15(6):902-906. doi: 10.1016/j.jsxm.2018.03.085. Epub 2018 Apr 26.

103. Opsomer D., Vyncke T., Mertens D., Ceulemans A., Claes KEY, Buncamper M., Monstrey S. "Fifteen-Year Experience with the Ghent Technique of Penile Inversion Vaginoplasty." *Plast Reconstr Surg.* 2021 Sep. 1 ; 148(3):416e-424e. PMID: 34432697.

used to line the walls of the neovagina. During these manipulations, the skin is used to form the wall of the vagina but loses much of its innervation and therefore its sensitivity. In the case of insufficient penile skin or after failure of a vaginoplasty by inversion, the use of a flap of peritoneum is a promising alternative[104]. The clitoris is reconstructed from the tissue of the glans, but the size of the glans is greatly reduced, also reducing its innervation and sensitivity.

In the USA, the operation costs at least $20,000, and in France between €7,000 and €15,000, which is 100 % refundable up to the health service reimbursement limit, provided that the person is recognised as having an ALD ("Affection de longue durée" or long-term condition) (whereas gender dysphoria is not considered an illness).
The neovagina has no natural cleaning or lubrication mechanism. Ongoing care is usually necessary after the operation and involves the use of a vaginal dilator, the aim of which is to stabilise or enlarge the cavity.
After vaginoplasty, if the patient follows the post-operative instructions (in particular regular exercise or sexual intercourse to maintain the space created to accommodate the vagina), a sexual partner may not notice the transformation undergone. However, it is advisable to inform them of this.
It is important to remember that the prostate remains in place to prevent urinary incontinence, and for this

104. Sachan A., Jain P., Sharma P., Goel V. "Male-to-Female Gender Affirmation Vaginoplasty via Laparoscopic Pedicled Peritoneal Flap-An Initial Experience." *Indian J Plast Surg.* 2022 Jul. 18 ; 55(2):211-215.

reason early diagnosis of prostate cancer should not be overlooked in trans women, even after complete surgery.

**Possible procedures to transform a woman into a trans man**

**Facial surgery:** to give a more masculine appearance by remodelling the chin to accentuate its angles, the jaws to increase their prominence using fillers, and the nose to reshape it.

**Thoracic surgery**: to remove both breasts.

**Genital surgery** to transform the genitals. Until 18 November 2016, removal of the uterus (hysterectomy) and ovaries (oophorectomy) was compulsory in France in order to register one's sex change officially. This removal avoided the risk of cancer from long-term hormone therapy.

There are two possible procedures for creating a phallus: **metoidioplasty** and **phalloplasty**.
Despite the complexity of phallus surgery as described below, we think it would be useful to detail it for those who might be interested, and above all to demonstrate to everyone the extreme precision required for this surgery, when "sex change" is presented as easy. No, it is not easy, and it is never satisfactory.

**Metoidioplasty** involves a vaginectomy, clitoral lengthening, urethral lengthening, scrotoplasty and bilateral implantation of testicular prostheses[105]. The vaginal mucosa is completely removed, except for a small area close to the native urethral meatus, which will later be used for urethroplasty. The vaginal vault is completely closed, creating a male-type perineum.

Clitoral degloving (it is turned inside out like a glove) is performed by a circular incision between the inner and outer layer of the clitoral hood down to the urethral plate, followed by partial or complete dissection of the suspensory ligaments to lengthen and straighten the clitoris, which had been enlarged beforehand through hormone therapy and sometimes the use of a vacuum device for a period of six months prior to surgery.

The most difficult part of the operation is the urethroplasty, which is essential if the patient wishes to be able to urinate standing up. It begins with the reconstruction of the bulbar urethra by joining the well-vascularised vaginal flap to the proximal part of the urethral plate. Additional reconstruction is performed by combining different available flaps and grafts (forearm, abdomen, thigh, leg).

When the urethral plate is long, urethral reconstruction can be achieved by simply tubularising the wide plate. If a urethral plate is insufficient, the remaining gap is covered with a buccal mucosa graft or a skin graft from the labia minora.

The size of the graft depends on the length of the new urethra. The abdominal part of the neourethra is created

105. Bordas N., Stojanovic B., Bizic M., Szanto A., Djordjevic M. L. "Metoidioplasty: Surgical Options and Outcomes in 813 Cases." *Front Endocrinol* (Lausanne). 2021 Oct. 13; 12: 760284. doi: 10.3389/fendo.2021.760284.

in the form of a flap made from the labia minora or a dorsal clitoral skin flap. The inner surface of one of the labia minora is dissected to the appropriate size to cover the dorsal part of the neourethra.
The pedicle is then mobilised and lengthened with the subcutaneous tissue of the labia majora to allow suturing with the dorsal part of the neourethra without tension. The urethra is calibrated to at least 16 gauge, and a silicone stent is placed in the neourethra to hydrate the inner surface and maintain the urethral calibre. The glans is opened on the midline by two parallel incisions, the two wings of the glans are then widely dissected and the neourethral meatus placed at the tip of the glans. The remaining skin of the clitoris and labia minora is used to cover the shaft of the penis. Scrotoplasty is then performed by joining the two labia majora on the midline and silicone testicular prostheses are implanted through bilateral incisions above the labia majora. In patients with an enlarged pubis, fatty tissue is resected to make urination safer in the standing position and to improve aesthetics.
This procedure, which takes an average of 3 to 5 hours, gives the genitals a masculine appearance, making it possible to urinate in an upright position and achieve a full erogenous sensation with sexual arousal, but without the possibility of intercourse with penetration, due to the small size of the neophallus.

**Phalloplasty** consists of constructing a penis using skin and tissue from the labia or other sources (free autografts from the forearm, thigh, latissimus dorsi[106] or abdomen). Autografts roll part of the skin over itself to build a neourethra, and another part outwards to prepare the neopenis skin, leaving these attached to the donor area to preserve their vascularisation. Once the preparation is complete, a catheter is used to support the neophallus before it is grafted to the pubic area and the procedure is usually completed with the construction of a scrotum using the skin and tissue of the labia which are then filled with testicular prostheses.

This is a long (4 to 10 hours, often involving two teams) and complex operation, which can cost up to €35,000 in France.

To ensure that the new penis is rigid, a penile prosthesis is included, with a pump to enable erection. The model - the mechanism and length of the penile implant - will be chosen according to anatomy.

The penile implant achieves rigidity by activating the pump which is usually located in the scrotum. The rigidity thus obtained makes sexual relations with penetration possible. This procedure can be carried out six months after the urethra has been constructed.

## Complications of this complex surgery

These long and difficult operations entail increased risks in cases of diabetes, obesity or blood circulation problems, either during anaesthesia or post-operatively. Candidates

106. Djordjevic M. L., Bencic M., Kojovic V., Stojanovic B., Bizic M., Kojic S., Krstic Z., Korac G. "Musculocutaneous latissimus dorsi flap for phalloplasty in female to male gender affirmation surgery." *World J Urol.* 2019 Apr.; 37(4):631-637. doi: 10.1007/s00345-019-02641-w. Epub 2019 Jan. 23. PMID: 30673829.

for this type of surgery must be carefully informed of these risks beforehand. Therapeutic education and close monitoring throughout the healing process are essential to support female patients who have become men, and to detect and treat these complications if necessary[107].

**Possible complications of masculinisation surgery**

Breast surgery is followed by complications in one-third of cases[108]. Both metoidioplasty[109] and phalloplasty run the risk of poor healing, infection, rejection and necrosis of the flap or infection of the prostheses[110].

The neourethra may shrink, become infected or develop diverticula. The prostheses required for erection may become infected, rupture or fail.

In the majority of reported cases, urethro-cutaneous fistula is the most common urethral complication, with an incidence ranging from 15 % to 70 %[111]. Jeffrey B. Frie-

107. Cristofari S., Bertrand B., Leuzzi S., Rem K., Rausky J., Revol M., Atlan M., Stivala A. "Postoperative complications of male to female sex reassignment surgery : A 10-year French retrospective study." *Ann Chir Plast Esthet.* 2019 Feb. ; 64(1):24-32.

108. Kääriäinen M., Salonen K., Helminen M., Karhunen-Enckell U. "Chest-wall contouring surgery in female-to-male transgender patients : A one-center retrospective analysis of applied surgical techniques and results." *Scand J Surg.* 2017 Mar. ; 106(1):74-79. Epub 2016 Jun. 23.

109. Stojanovic B., Djordjevic M. L. "Updates on metoidioplasty." *Neurourol Urodyn.* 2023 Jun. ; 42(5):956-962. doi : 10.1002/nau.25102. Epub 2022 Nov. 20. PMID : 36403289.

110. Briles B. L., Middleton R. Y., Celtik K. E., Crane C. N., Safir M., Santucci R. A. "Penile Prosthesis Placement by a Dedicated Transgender Surgery Unit : A Retrospective Analysis of Complications." *J Sex Med.* 2022 Apr. 1 ; 19(4):641-649.

111. Fascelli M., Sajadi K. P., Dugi D. D., Dy GW. "Urinary symptoms after genital gender-affirming penile construction, urethral lengthening and vaginectomy." *Transl Androl Urol.* 2023 May 31 ; 12(5):932-943. doi : 10.21037/tau-22-675. Epub 2023 Mar. 1.

drich and colleagues, analysing the results of fifty studies[112] of phalloplasty, estimate the incidence to be close to 40 %.

**Possible complications of feminising surgery**

Vaginoplasty is followed by complications in more than one-third of cases[113][114]. These can occur early or late, and be haemorrhagic, cosmetic or functional in nature. They may affect all the anatomical parts reconstructed : vagina, urethra, clitoris, labia minora and majora. In exceptional cases, these complications may even lead to death[115].

Vaginoplasty can be complicated by sores of the rectum, bladder or urinary tract, which sometimes develop into chronic fistulas[116]. An urethrovaginal fistula (1.5 % of cases) means that urine is evacuated through the vagina

112. Remington A. C., Morrison S. D., Massie J. P., Crowe C. S., Shakir A., Wilson S. C., Vyas K. S. , Lee G. K., Friedrich J. B. "Outcomes after Phalloplasty : Do Transgender Patients and Multiple Urethral Procedures Carry a Higher Rate of Complication ?" *Plast Reconstr Surg.* 2018 Feb. ; 141(2):220e-229e.

113. Dreher P. C., Edwards D., Hager S., Dennis M., Belkoff A., Mora J., Tarry S., Rumer K. L. "Complications of the neovagina in male-to-female transgender surgery : A systematic review and meta-analysis with discussion of management." *Clin Anat.* 2018 Mar. ; 31(2):191-199. doi : 10.1002/ca.23001. Epub 2017 Nov. 10. PMID : 29057562.

114. Ferrando CA. "Vaginoplasty Complications." *Clin Plast Surg.* 2018 Jul. ; 45(3):361-368. doi : 10.1016/j.cps.2018.03.007. Epub 2018 Mar. 31. PMID : 29908624.

115. Negenborn V. L., van der Sluis W. B., Meijerink W. J. H. J., Bouman M. B. "Lethal Necrotizing Cellulitis Caused by ESBL-Producing E. Coli after Laparoscopic Intestinal Vaginoplasty." *J Pediatr Adolesc Gynecol.* 2017 Feb. ; 30(1):e19-e21. Epub 2016 Sep. 21. PMID : 27664856.

116. Pansritum K., Thomrongdullaphak S., Suwajo P., "A Rectoprostatic Fascia Reinforcement Flap for Rectal Injury and Rectoneovaginal Fistula in Gender-Affirmation Surgery." *Plast Reconstr Surg.* 2022 Oct. 1 ; 150(4):909-913. Epub 2022 Aug. 4.

during urination. A vaginorectal fistula (1.5 % of cases) results in stools being passed through the vagina during defecation and requires further surgery.
Haemorrhage from the surgical site frequently arises from spongy remnants behind the urethral mucosa and around the urinary meatus.
Fever accompanied by a purulent vaginal discharge is indicative of a vaginal infection (almost 10 %), while cloudy urine is indicative of a urinary and/or prostate infection (1.6 %).
Most postoperative healing problems happen to the pelvic floor, often requiring specialised care[117]. Urinary retention in the bladder when the urinary catheter is removed requires the catheter to be replaced in almost 4 % of cases. The skin lining of the neovagina may turn inside out when the flexible conformer is removed.
Pain and urinary tract infection are the main complaints. In the medium and long term, the neovagina tends to shrink (17.8 %) in depth and diameter, even if it is frequently penetrated. Vaginoplasty must therefore always be followed by regular dilatation sessions for life using rigid dilators.
Having a vagina lined with skin rather than mucous membrane offers no protection against sexually transmitted infections : mycoses, condylomata (HPV), chlamydia, syphilis, herpes and HIV, all of which means the use of condoms is required.

---

117. Jiang D. D., Gallagher S., Burchill L., Berli J., Dugi D 3rd. "Implementation of a Pelvic Floor Physical Therapy Program for Transgender Women Undergoing Gender-Affirming Vaginoplasty." Obstet Gynecol. 2019 May; 133(5):1003-1011. doi: 10.1097/AOG.0000000000003236. PMID: 30969210.

**Many disappointments after an irreversible transition**

Surgical interventions lead to irreversible mutilation, often with questionable aesthetic results and unsatisfactory function[118] [119] [120].

For trans women, current techniques have not fully achieved the ideal goal of reconstructing genitalia that resemble female genitalia in full form and function (known as cis-female genitalia).

Trans men can only achieve an erection with a penile implant and a pump system and suffer from a lack of tactile sensation on the neophallus.

The skin of a trans woman's neovagina is not very sensitive and there is a risk of progressive and permanent shrinkage.

Some people bitterly regret this, as they themselves admit. They speak of a "one-way transition highway", on which they were rushed at full speed without any consideration for their family's views, or even the opinion of a psychologist or doctor.

How can a child assess the consequences of permanent loss of fertility and abnormal or at least unsatisfactory

118. De Vries, A., McGuire, T., Steensma, E., Wagenaar, T., Doreleijers, P. & Cohen-Kettenis, P. (2014). *Résultat psychologique du jeune adulte après suppression de la puberté et changement de sexe.*

119. Kerckhof M. E., Kreukels B. P. C., Nieder T. O., Becker-Hébly I., van de Grift T. C., Staphorsius A. S., Köhler A., Heylens G., Elaut E. "Prevalence of Sexual Dysfunctions in Transgender Persons: Results from the ENIGI Follow-Up Study." *J Sex Med.* 2019 Dec.; 16(12):2018-2029. doi: 10.1016/j.jsxm.2019.09.003. Epub 2019 Oct. 24. Erratum in: *J Sex Med.* 2020 Apr.; 17(4):830. PMID: 31668732.

120. Bishop M. D., Morgan-Daniel J., Alappattu M. J. "Pain and Dysfunction Reported After Gender-Affirming Surgery: A Scoping Review." *Phys Ther.* 2023 Jul. 1; 103(7).

sexual relations? Some people would like to go back to the way things were and are known as "detransitioners"[121]. They have not found the solution to their problems; they realise that they have made a mistake and often say that they have been deceived[122 123].
Unfortunately for them, surgical transformations are irreversible.
This would be enough to justify the ban that should be in place on modifying a child's body, such as the removal of breasts currently authorised at the age of 16 in France with parental consent.
Some, such as Chloe Cole[124 125] in the USA and Keira Bell[126] in the UK, have taken legal action.
"I was an unhappy girl who needed help. Instead, I was treated like an experiment." "As I matured, I recognised that gender dysphoria was a symptom of my overall misery, not its cause. Five years after beginning my medical transition to becoming male, I began the process of detransitioning." [127]

---

121. https://www.marianne.net/agora/tribunes-libres/transgenrisme-de-jeunes-detransitionneurs-viennent-nous-apporter-le-recit-de-leur-parcours
122. https://fr.aleteia.org/2022/05/24/ces-enfants-qui-regrettent-leur-changement-de-sexe/
123. https://www.lefigaro.fr/actualite-france/la-detresse-de-ces-jeunes-qui-regrettent-d-avoir-voulu-changer-de-sexe-20220530
124. https://www.theblaze.com/news/detransitioner-chloe-cole-sues-hospital
125. https://nypost.com/2023/07/27/detransitioner-tells-congress-her-childhood-was-ruined-by-gender-reassignment/
126. https://tradfem.wordpress.com/2021/04/13/keira-bell-mon-corps-ne-tait-pas-le-probleme/
127. Keira Bell, telling her story *Persuasion.* https://www.persuasion.community/p/keira-bell-my-story

A study by Swedish trans activists of 2,679 people[128] had claimed that medical transition would have a positive effect on the quality of life and mental health of transgender people. But another Swedish study has concluded that, on the contrary, after a sex change, trans people have significantly higher risks of mortality, suicidal behaviour and psychiatric morbidity than the general population. This study suggests that sex reassignment, although it alleviates gender dysphoria (at least temporarily), may not be sufficient as a treatment for gender dysphoria and should prompt improvements in the psychological and/or psychiatric and somatic care for this group of patients[129].
As a result, in 2023, the Karolinska Hospital, a world pioneer in gender surgery, decided to stop performing it on minors[130], citing the lack of evidence for the effectiveness of these treatments in improving the well-being of patients, and the dangerous side-effects of the drugs.
In the UK, the paediatric department of the Tavistock clinic, after pioneering transition programmes for minors, has just abandoned[131] them under pressure from

128. Bränström R., Pachankis J. E. "Reduction in Mental Health Treatment Utilization Among Transgender Individuals After Gender-Affirming Surgeries: A Total Population Study." *Am J Psychiatry.* 2020 Aug. 1; 177(8):727-734 Epub 2019 Oct. 4. Erratum in: *Am J Psychiatry.* 2020 Aug 1; 177(8):734
129. Dhejne C., Lichtenstein P., Boman M., Johansson A. L., Långström N., Landén M. "Long-term follow-up of transsexual persons undergoing sex reassignment surgery: cohort study in Sweden." *PLoS One.* 2011 Feb. 22; 6(2):e16885. doi: 10.1371/journal.pone.0016885
130. *RTS* 28 juin 2023, "La Suède freine sur la question du changement de sexe des mineurs." https://www.rts.ch/info/monde/12295658-la-suede-freine-sur-la-question-du-changement-de-sexe-des-mineurs.html
131. https://www.lavie.fr/actualite/societe/enfants-transgenres-pourquoi-la-clinique-tavistock-va-fermer-en-angleterre-83876.php

the health authorities following an independent audit[132]. A psychiatrist in charge of child protection had reported serious abuses in the care of children to her superiors, and in return had been harassed by them. She was finally awarded £20,000 in damages[133] by the Tavistock clinic.

Articles reporting on single-centre series written by trans activists, doctors[134] and surgeons who make a living from this activity are always full of praise[135][136][137][138][139] and high-

132. https://www.bbc.com/news/uk-56539466

133. https://www.genethique.org/identite-de-genre-des-dommages-et-interets-pour-une-psychiatre-en-charge-de-la-protection-des-enfants/

134. Arnoldussen M., van der Miesen A. I. R., Elzinga W. S., Alberse A. E., Popma A., Steensma T. D., de Vries A. L. C. "Self-Perception of Transgender Adolescents After Gender-Affirming Treatment : A Follow-Up Study into Young Adulthood." *LGBT Health.* 2022 May-Jun. ; 9(4):238-246 Epub 2022 Apr. 26.

135. "Male-to-Female Gender-Affirming Surgery : 20-Year Review of Technique and Surgical Results." https://www.frontiersin.org/articles/10.3389/fsurg.2021.639430/full

136. Wiepjes C. M., Nota N. M., de Blok C. J. M., Klaver M., de Vries A. L. C., Wensing-Kruger S. A., de Jongh R. T., Bouman M. B., Steensma T. D., Cohen-Kettenis P., Gooren L. J. G., Kreukels B. P. C., den Heijer M. "The Amsterdam Cohort of Gender Dysphoria Study (1972-2015) : Trends in Prevalence, Treatment, and Regrets." *J Sex Med.* 2018 Apr. ; 15(4):582-590. Epub 2018 Feb 17.

137. Park R. H., Liu Y. T., Samuel A., Gurganus M., Gampper T. J., Corbett S. T., Shahane A., Stranix J. T. "Long-term Outcomes After Gender-Affirming Surgery : 40-Year Follow-up Study." *Ann Plast Surg.* 2022 Oct. 1 ; 89(4):431-436.

138. Papadopulos N. A., Ehrenberger B., Zavlin D., Lellé J. D., Henrich G., Kovacs L., Herschbach P., Machens H. G., Schaff J. "Quality of Life and Satisfaction in Transgender Men After Phalloplasty in a Retrospective Study." *Ann Plast Surg.* 2021 Jul. 1 ; 87(1):91-97.

139. Wu S. H., Shen B. H., Perng C. K., Wang T. H., Shih Y. C., Ma H., Wu H. Y. "Complications of free-flap procedures for phalloplasty in female-to-male transgender surgery : 25-year experience a single medical center." *J Chin Med Assoc.* 2022 Mar. 1 ; 85(3):341-345.

light the superiority of their personal technique, but the sheer number of these techniques (phalloplasty using a flap from the forearm, abdomen, greater dorsalis or labia majora, etc.), the lack of consensus on the best one[140] and the numerous macro-analyses[141][142][143] highlighting the considerable biases of these studies show that these problems have not been resolved.

A review of over 100 international medical studies of transgender people who had undergone surgery, by the University of Birmingham's Aggressive Research Intelligence Facility (ARIF) concluded that it was not possible to say categorically that surgery improves the mental health[144] of transexuals, some of whom remain depressed and even suicidal after the operation.

Overall, the results do not usually live up to the initial expectations of trans people and sometimes lead to legal

140. Al-Tamimi M., Pigot G. L., Elfering L., Özer M., de Haseth K., van de Grift T. C., Mullender M. G., Bouman M. B., Van der Sluis W. B. "Genital Gender-Affirming Surgery in Transgender Men in The Netherlands from 1989 to 2018: The Evolution of Surgical Care." *Plast Reconstr Surg.* 2020 Jan.; 145(1):153e-161e

141. Oles N., Darrach H., Landford W., Garza M., Twose C., Park C. S., Tran P., Schechter L. S., Lau B., Coon D. "Gender Affirming Surgery: A Comprehensive, Systematic Review of All Peer-reviewed Literature and Methods of Assessing Patient-centered Outcomes (Part 1: Breast/Chest, Face, and Voice)." *Ann Surg.* 2022 Jan. 1; 275(1):e52-e66.

142. Dunford C., Bell K., Rashid T. "Genital Reconstructive Surgery in Male to Female Transgender Patients: A Systematic Review of Primary Surgical Techniques, Complication Profiles, and Functional Outcomes from 1950 to Present Day." *Eur Urol Focus.* 2021 Mar.; 7(2):464-471. doi: 10.1016/j.euf.2020.01.004. Epub 2020 Feb. 13.

143. Patel H., Arruarana V., Yao L., Cui X., Ray E. "Effects of hormones and hormone therapy on breast tissue in transgender patients: a concise review." *Endocrine.* 2020 Apr.; 68(1):6-15. Epub 2020 Feb. 17.

144. "Sex changes are not effective, say researchers." https://www.theguardian.com/society/2004/jul/30/health.mentalhealth

complaints[145] and disappointments[146], which can even increase the risk of suicide[147]. In countries where these procedures have been authorised for children[148], there are increasing reports of people regretting the sex change they underwent at an early age.

In 2021, Dr Lisa Littman published the results of an online survey of gender detransitioners, 40 % of whom said that their gender dysphoria was caused by a mental health problem and 62 % of whom felt that health professionals had not investigated whether psychological trauma was a factor in their decisions to transition[149].

**Why should this so-called "cosmetic" surgery be available free on the health service?** [150]

Sex-change operations are irreversible and require lifelong treatment and medication. But even though gender dysphoria is no longer considered an illness and is therefore cosmetic surgery for convenience, it is 100 % refundable by the French health service[151], unlike den-

145. Like Keira Bell in the UK. https://www.causeur.fr/keira-bell-justice-royaume-uni-transgenre-189864
146. https://www.marianne.net/agora/tribunes-libres/transgenrisme-de-jeunes-detransitionneurs-viennent-nous-apporter-le-recit-de-leur-parcours
147. https://nouveau-monde.ca/devenir-trans-mene-trop-souvent-au-suicide-informez-familles-et-candidats-pour-leur-securite/
148. https://www.juristespourlenfance.com/2021/03/25/je-pensais-que-je-tais-transgenre-temoignages-de-detransitionneurs/
149. https://nypost.com/2022/06/18/detransitioned-teens-explain-why-they-regret-changing-genders/
150. While women who have a complex about their large breasts have to pay for this surgery, which is often not purely cosmetic.
151. This seems to be a worldwide exception, apart from in a few Democratic States since the Biden Act, however even there the costs involved are not entirely covered as they are in France.

tal care, glasses and hearing aids that relieve real medical conditions. Why is this?
In major medical centres you will find the name of surgeons who inspire confidence and who perform sexual mutilations on minors: mastectomies will often be presented by euphemisms such as "torsoplasty" or "top surgery", or castrations labelled "bottom surgery" (whereby trans vocabulary is taken up by professional doctors).
These surgeries are authorised in France for anyone under the age of 18, with parental consent, and are carried out in private clinics in Paris and the rest of the country[152].

In its press release of 25 February 2022, the French Academy of Medicine drew attention to the issue of medically treating minors for gender dysphoria[153]:

> "While in France the use of hormone blockers or hormones of the opposite sex is allowed with parental authorisation and without age restrictions, the greatest of care is required with this usage, given the side effects such as the impact on growth, the risk of increased bone fragility and sterility, the emotional and cognitive consequences and, for girls, the onset of symptoms reminiscent of the menopause."[...]
>
> "As for surgical treatments, in particular mastectomies authorised in France from the age of 14,

152. https://www.observatoirepetitesirene.org/
153. https://www.academie-medecine.fr/la-medecine-face-a-la-transidentite-de-genre-chez-les-enfants-et-les-adolescents/Publié le 25 février 2022

and those involving the external genital tract (vulva, penis), it should be emphasised that they are irreversible."

# 4.
# Psychological and psychiatric consequences of promoting trans identity

Contrary to the purely political opinion of the UN[154], which hopes in this way to reduce the discrimination felt by transsexuals, Dr McHugh, chief psychiatrist at the Johns Hopkins hospital, points out that transgenderism is a mental disorder. *Changing sex is biologically impossible*[155].

These people need psychological care, and states such as California, New Jersey, and Massachusetts, which have denied the medical aspect of the problem and made it so that people no longer have to consult a psychiatrist before undergoing any medical or surgical procedure,

154. "WHO removes 'gender identity disorder' from its list of medical conditions, a victory for transgender activists" https://news.un.org/fr/story/2019/05/1044591

155. Dr McHugh, psychiatrist at Johns Hopkins: "Transgenderism is a 'mental disorder'; changing sex is 'biologically impossible'". https://ifamnews.com/fr/psychiatre-de-johns-hopkins-le-transgenre-est-un-trouble-mental-le-changement-de-sexe-est-biologiquement-impossible

have in practice encouraged this mental disorder. “I’m absolutely convinced that this is folly and it’s going to collapse”, says Paul McHugh, former head of Psychiatry at Johns Hopkins, who is now very old and therefore considered a “has-been”.

But of course, Western lobbies have been so effective that it is now forbidden even to think this, let alone write it, on pain of being branded transphobic[156] and taken to court.

So, let’s take a humble look at the opinions of a few psychiatrists in this field and their published data[157].

In her article “Reading the difference between the sexes”[158], psychoanalyst Marie Balmary writes that this difference is a constitutive part of the individual: “*The emergence of the subject only takes place in relation to another subject different from itself*”, adding that “*the difference between the sexes appears as the primary model - the paradigm - of all other situations of otherness*”. She adds that “*gender difference is a good thing for children*, it gives them balance.”

In his book *Sex Aequo, le quiproquo des sexes*, psychiatrist and neuropsychologist Jean-Paul Mialet expresses concern about the trend towards gender undifferentiation:

156. As is the case for the head of the Hungarian state, for example.
157. Cf. “Théorie du genre: les enfants pourraient en souffrir selon les […]” – par Lise Caillaud, 5 mars 2014, Théorie du genre (theoriedugenre.fr): ” We note that it was still allowed in 2014 to broach this subject, even in disagreement with the prevailing thinking.
158. Marie Balmary, « Lire la différence des sexes », *Projet*, 2005/4 n° 287, p. 23-29.

> "Very early on, differences become apparent. We must not forget that consciousness is formed in the experience of the body's interactions with the environment: two different bodies lead to distinct states of consciousness, and we can say that consciousness is gendered, like the body."[159][160]

In his view, the difference between the sexes is fundamental to everyone's identity: we define ourselves in opposition to others and "*the difference between the sexes is a fundamental otherness*". This "*pedestal of differences*" is necessary for the development of the child:

> "The child will later develop a conscious desire to be closer to the camp to which he or she belongs. We want to be like Mum or Dad".

And let's add, not like "parent 1" or "parent 2", it is by this kind of shortcut that we measure the folly of "men"[161].

Catherine Chabert[162], psychoanalyst from Descartes University in Paris, shares a similar opinion to her colleague, and advocates respect for differences, which are rich in reference points. For her, and contrary to received ideas and intellectual orthodoxy:

---

159. http://leplus.nouvelobs.com/contribution/204206-la-difference-entre-hommes-et-femmes-est-elle-une-question-d-education.html
160. http://www.lexpress.fr/culture/livre/jean-paul-mialet-et-sa-vision-a-contre-courant-des-differences-hommes-femmes_980947.html
161. Which, in academic parlance, means men AND women!
162. Author of *L'amour de la différence* (PUF, 2011).

> "The difference between the sexes fosters social cohesion. Conversely, uniformity and sameness would lead to narcissism, which is detrimental to living in society".

She returns to the obsession with equality of the self-righteous Left. But by trying to erase differences, these ideologues have created a whole host of new ones, from which it will be very difficult to extricate ourselves. The psychiatrist would like people to understand that:

> "Equality has nothing to do with being identical [...] It's very important that the fundamental differences between men and women, and between fathers and mothers, are marked. Differences make it possible to look elsewhere for what one person has not given but another can offer; they make allowances for discrepancies and disappointments and combat the deleterious excesses of idealisation".

Another doctor of psychology, Dr Leonard Sax[163], concurs:

> "As far as children are concerned, the difference between the sexes is necessary and constitutive of each person's identity: "by concealing these distinctions between the sexes, we harm the child. At home and at school, they feel misunderstood, abandoned and left to fend for themselves".[164]

163. Read *Why Gender Matters: What Parents and Teachers Need to Know about the Emerging Science of Sex Difference, Doubleday, 2005; revised edition published in 2017.*

164. http://www.lexpress.fr/actualite/societe/nier-ce-qui-distingue-les-sexes-nuit-a-l-enfant_1314273.html

This last remark is very important, because it is a source of the depression, isolation and unease that are looming. The current tendency is to interpret any trouble as "gender dysphoria" when the child is simply abandoned in the name of current fashions that have become dogma. We can imagine that the additional suffering caused by the isolation resulting from the absurd and pointless lockdowns can only have aggravated the precarious situation of these children, glued to their screens, the only contact allowed … and favoured by TikTok lobbyists or other powerful players.
Among other things, Dr Sax recounts an experiment by Yale University researchers on stereotypes, which it is claimed are pure social constructs[165] :

> They placed trucks and dolls in front of young monkeys, primates that do not know the masculine/feminine character of these objects. However, a large majority of males chose the trucks.

The obvious retort will be that we are not monkeys. However, the forty-something and slightly older generations have clearly understood that the attractions of toys are socially constructed… They're wrong.

165. The Collapse of Parenting: How We Hurt Our Kids When We Treat Them Like Grown-Ups (2015), Dr Leonard Sax

# 5.
# Sex reassignment treatments do not protect transgender people from suicide

One of the main arguments given to parents to get them to accept their child's desire for transition is that it will prevent their child from committing suicide. This is a lie with serious consequences, as demonstrated by the data (already referred to) from the Amsterdam gender dysphoria treatment clinic, which found that the overall mortality rate of their treated patients was double that of non-trans, and that the risk of suicide "*has not increased*" after five decades of treatment.

**The suicidal tendency of transgender people is high, regardless of the country in which they live**

In Great Britain, the Biley study[166] involving 889 trans people revealed a lifetime prevalence of 84 % of suicidal

166. Bailey, L., Ellis, S., et McNeil, J. (2014). "Suicide risk in the UK trans population and the role of gender transitioning in decreasing suicidal ideation and suicide attempt." *Mental Health Review Journal*, 19(4), pages 209 à 220. http://doi.org/10.1108/MHRJ-05-2014-0015

thoughts and 48 % of suicide attempts. In Ontario[167], in a single year, 35.1 % of trans people seriously considered committing suicide and 11.2 % actually did so.

In Thailand[168], out of 411 LGBTQ+ participants, 39 % reported having had suicidal thoughts in their lifetime, 19.0 % suicidal thoughts in the last twelve months and 13.1 % suicide attempts in their lifetime.

The North American Austin study[169] indicates that 82 % of transgender people have felt suicidal and 40 % have attempted suicide, with suicidal tendency being highest among young people. The Trevor Project[170] studying the experiences of nearly 35,000 LGBTQ+ Americans aged between 13 and 24 confirms these exorbitant suicide rates and attempts to determine what could reduce them.
The Spanish study by Elena García-Vega[171] evalu-

167. Bauer, G., Schiem, A., Travers, R. et Hammond, R. (2015b). "Intervenable factors associated with suicide risk in transgender persons: A respondent driven suicide risk sampling study in Ontario, Canada." *BMC Public Health.* doi: 10.1186/s12889-015-1867-2 http://doi. org/10.1186/s12889-015-1867-2

168. Kittiteerasack P., Matthews A. K., Steffen A., Corte C., McCreary L. L., Bostwick W., Park C., Johnson T. P. "The influence of minority stress on indicators of suicidality among lesbian, gay, bisexual and transgender adults in Thailand." *J Psychiatr Ment Health Nurs.* 2021 Aug.; 28(4):656-669. doi: 10.1111/jpm.12713. Epub 2020 Dec. 1. PMID: 33190351.

169. Austin A., Craig S. L., D'Souza S., McInroy L. B. "Suicidality Among Transgender Youth: Elucidating the Role of Interpersonal Risk Factors." *J Interpers Violence.* 2022 Mar.; 37(5-6):NP2696-NP2718. Epub 2020 Apr. 29.

170. https://www.thetrevorproject.org/resources/article/facts-about-lgbtq-youth-suicide/

171. García-Vega E., Camero A., Fernández M., Villaverde A. "Suicidal ideation and suicide attempts in persons with gender dysphoria." *Psicothema.* 2018 Aug.; 30(3):283-288. doi: 10.7334/psicothema2017.438. https://pubmed.ncbi.nlm.nih.gov/30009750/

ates suicidal thoughts at 48.3 % and suicidal acts at 23.8 %.

Overall, transsexuals are 4 to 6 times more suicide-prone than other sexual minorities (homosexuals, lesbians and bisexuals) and 10 to 20 times more than heterosexuals.

**Proportion of Adults Who Have Attempted Suicide**

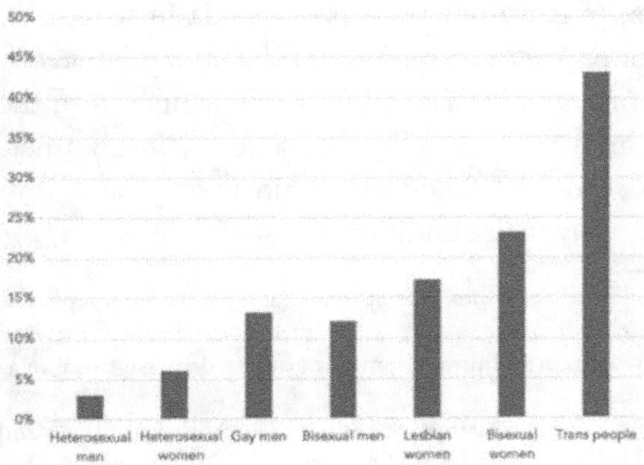


*Source: "A systematic review and meta-analysis of disparities in the prevalence of suicide ideation and attempt among bisexual populations," Archives of Sexual Behavior, 2019; "Suicidality among trans people in Ontario: implications for social work and social justice," Service Social, 2013.*

This very high risk of suicide among transsexuals, as well as the frequency of self-harm and drug use, is a serious health problem that needs to be taken into account in order to provide the most appropriate response possible.

## Transsexuals' derogatory rights

In a classic attempt to portray minorities as victims, trans activists claim that these suicides have nothing to do with their particular psychological state, sexual orientation or

gender identity, but only with the stress of being a minority and the social mistreatment they experience.
This has enabled them to obtain special rights that are often considerable, such as the right to change their first name and sex on their identity card simply by declaring their gender, to accuse those who call them by the name given to them at birth of transphobia and to take legal action against them, to use the toilets and changing rooms normally reserved for the other sex, to carry out trans propaganda in schools[172], to benefit from a "*better reception of LGBTQ+ asylum seekers and refugees in France*"[173] and an over-representation in the media[174], in movies[175], in television series[176], in commercials[177][178], in schools[179][180] and in certain theme parks[181] in order to downplay their condition.

---

172. https://habilomedias.ca/sites/default/files/lesson-plans/lecon_representations_transgenres.pdf

173. https://www.egalite-femmes-hommes.gouv.fr/droits-lgbt-et-relations-internationales

174. According to the Association of Lesbian, Gay, Bisexual, Trans and Intersex Journalists, trans-identity is "finally being seen as a news story in its own right". https://www.radiofrance.fr/franceinter/podcasts/la-chronique-mediatique/la-chronique-mediatique-de-cyril-lacarriere-du-mardi-04-avril-2023-2111093

175. https://www.senscritique.com/liste/Courts_metrages_LGBT/879836

176. https://www.rtl.fr/actu/debats-societe/avec-les-series-tele-les-transgenres-gagnent-en-visibilite-7778982296

177. http://fastncurious.fr/2016/11/21/14341/

178. https://www.radiofrance.fr/franceinter/promue-par-une-influenceuse-transgenre-une-biere-budweiser-boycottee-par-les-conservateurs-americains-3691015

179.https://www.revuedesdeuxmondes.fr/ecole-trans-education-nationale/

180. https://www.famillechretienne.fr/40529/article/polemique-apres-la-tenue-dun-atelier-de-propagande-trans-a-lecole-alsacienne

181. On 28 March 2022, Disney Group Chairwoman Karey Burke said she wanted more LGBTQ+ and racial minority characters in lead roles in studio productions (up to 50 % of the cast) and romance between characters of the same gender.

Yet the discrimination they suffer is no different from that suffered by all other sexual minorities who do not have these derogatory rights and who commit suicide 4 to 6 times less often. This victimisation, orchestrated by the trans lobbies and associations, can only lock them into this painful status and can in no way help them out of their metaphysical issues.

**Possible reasons for the very high rate of transgender suicides**

The suicide of trans people could be linked in part to their extreme minority situation (minority stress). The number of adults over the age of 45 who identify themselves as transgender has remained stable in recent decades. In the USA, where they are most numerous, they represent 0.6 % of people aged 13 and over, of whom 38.5 % identify themselves as transgender women, 35.9 % as transgender men and 25.6 % as gender non-conforming. The percentage of trans people falls rapidly with age, from 1.43 % in the 13-17 age group to 0.45 % in the 25-45 age group and 0.32 % in the 65+ age group. Life experience therefore leads more than 80 % of teenagers who thought they were transgender to realise in adulthood that they were not, and to recognise themselves, for the most part, as gay or bisexual.

This "minority stress" is certainly not the main cause of the suicide risk for trans people, as other sexual minorities (gay, lesbian, bi) who are just as exposed to it commit suicide far less frequently.

What's more, there is little we can do about this minority stress other than to use psychological care to help trans people accept that they are a tiny minority, to accept themselves, to learn not to isolate themselves from others, to abandon their victim attitude, not to see transphobia everywhere for them to denounce, and to stop taking legal action against any non-trans people who talk about their issue. Other sexual minorities have been aware of this for a long time, and this could explain why they are much better integrated and more at ease.

The suicide of trans people reflects their intrinsic malaise, as shown by the fact that in a Danish study, the proportion of people with psychiatric problems was 6 times higher among transgender people (42.9 %) than in the rest of the population (7.1 %)[182]: a higher incidence of attention deficit, eating disorders and autism. These disorders, which they have experienced since they were young, have often been wrongly attributed to gender dysphoria by a medical and social community that is currently very oriented towards this, and are therefore not taken into account.

Adolescence and its bodily transformations raise legitimate questions, concerns and even anxieties in many children, particularly about sex and their sexual organs. At this age, they are very receptive and, if they come into contact with trans influencers and activists at school or on the Internet, or if they consult treatment providers, they can be persuaded that it is their sexual identity that is troubling them and that they should change it, exposing them to lifelong hormone treatments and irreversible mutilating surgery.

182. Erlangsen A., Jacobsen A. L., Ranning A., Delamare A. L., Nordentoft M., Frisch M. "Transgender Identity and Suicide Attempts and Mortality in Denmark." *JAMA*. 2023; 329(24):2145–2153. doi: 10.1001/jama.2023.8627

Social network influencers[183] and transgender support groups seem to play a major role in the "current epidemic" of young people who suddenly overnight find themselves in a class with three or four trans people[184].

**The unhappiness of trans people is also strongly linked to their self-perpetuating isolation**

Feeling, and even more so declaring oneself to be trans, tends to make contact with others less desirable, more difficult and rarer. But we are beings of emotion[185] more than we are rational or reflective beings. Contact with others, like living with a partner, improves our mood, soothes us, reduces stress and the risk of suicide, relieves tension and reinforces the feeling of being understood and accepted. Feeling different often dissuades trans people from reaching out to others and benefiting from these contacts, confining them to the trans community and leading them to brood about their condition, aggravating depression and the risk of suicide.

A survey on life satisfaction carried out by BMC Public Health shows that only 7.4 % of binary transgender people consider themselves to be satisfied, compared with 17.9 % of non-binary transgender people, 38 % of women and 40.6 % of men, confirming the considerable unease experienced by trans people.

---

183. Including those approached by ideologues and/or purveyors of lucrative interventions.

184. *Mauvais genre – une épidémie mondiale*, the first ever documentary critical of gender ideology.

185. The media and the ruling powers are well aware of this!

**Transgender people's unease may be exacerbated by complications and the often-disappointing results of medication and surgery**

Initially, asserting one's trans gender can be a source of relief for the individual, as they become part of a community that understands them. But the long, complicated and expensive transsexual physical transformation[186] involves an arduous route which questions the merits of this approach.

It requires lifelong hormone treatment, which, like any other treatment, can lead to complications[187]. Blocking testosterone can lead to osteoporosis (and the risk of fractures), cardiovascular problems, and worsen depression, increasing the risk of suicide in some patients. Conversely, virilising hormones can promote a state of pathological excitement or a psychotic episode[188].

Numerous surgical procedures lead to irreversible mutilation, sometimes with questionable aesthetic results, and a function that is often far removed from the hopes raised. We need only think of the suffering of trans men, who can only achieve an erection using a pump system, and the lack of tactile sensation in their neophallus. Trans women are often disheartened by the insensitivity and dryness of their neovaginal skin, and the risk of progressive shrinkage, which means they have to use vaginal dilators for the rest of their lives.

---

186. The fact that the costs of hormone-assisted sex reassignment surgery are fully covered by the French social security system is a worldwide anomaly that is difficult to justify, since it is accepted that it is not an illness.
187. Cf. dedicated chapter.
188. « Il faut bannir traitements hormonaux et bloqueurs de puberté, à visée transgenre chez les mineurs » – Docteur Nicole Delépine (nicoledelepine.fr)

Overall, the results are usually less than hoped for, and the disappointment that frequently results can exacerbate depression and the desire for suicide. In countries where these procedures have been authorised, there are increasing reports of people regretting the sex change they underwent at an early age.

In 2019, British science journalist Charlie Evans set up the "Detransition Advocacy Network", which in the space of three months received more than 300 messages from young people regretting their transition.

A macro-analysis of more than 100 international medical studies of transgender people operated on by the University of Birmingham concluded that it was not possible to give an opinion on the effectiveness of surgery on the mental health of transgender people, with some of them remaining depressed and even suicidal after the operation.

**How can we reduce the risk of suicide among young people who believe they suffer from gender dysphoria?**

To help them, the first thing to do is to reassure them that their worries about sexual matters are common at their age and that they disappear in over 80 % of cases when they reach adulthood.

Remind them that their parents, or other family members such as siblings or grandparents, love them and are there to help, whatever their problems.

If the anxieties persist, they should be referred to a neutral psychologist (neither anti nor pro-trans, and courageous enough not to submit to the dominant transgender-affirmative doctrine).

Audits by the Karolinska Institute in Stockholm[189] or the Tavistock Clinic in Birmingham[190] have shown that the specialist services to which children likely to be suffering from gender dysphoria are automatically referred are usually run by gender theory ideologues who are all too ready to confirm the diagnosis of dysphoria, without any serious medical or psychiatric examination, and to organise emergency treatment (hormonal treatment followed by surgery, etc.). It is essential to seek out professionals who are objective, non-partisan and "non-specialised", and to reject the notion of urgency. On the contrary, such serious decisions should be carefully thought through. But business is business!

And if the desire for transformation persists, they need to be objectively informed of the modalities and duration of the medical treatments, and of the burdensome and irreversible nature of the surgery. Knowing that you will in fact be transformed into a lifelong patient requiring hormonal treatments and medical monitoring until the end of your life, and agreeing to sacrifice your fertility, is a difficult but essential step if the "patient" is not to be disappointed by the discovery of reality.

The love of family and friends, complete information for teenagers without taboos and, if necessary, support from a non-partisan psychologist are the best ways of preventing teenage anguish and the delusions of the dominant transsexual propaganda, and of reducing the considerable risk of suicide that threatens transgender people.

---

189. https://www.ieb-eib.org/fr/actualite/statut-du-corps-humain/genre-et-sexualite/dysphorie-de-genre-la-suede-remet-en-question-les-traitements-hormonaux-sur-adolescents-2030.html?backto=bulletin

190. https://www.courrierinternational.com/article/transidentite-la-clinique-tavistock-recit-d-un-scandale-medical-britannique

# 6.
# Transgender and sports, inclusion or equity?

This chapter deals with a hotly debated issue, marked by sometimes impassioned positions. For this reason, we will concentrate on the facts, the indisputable facts, citing the opinions of certain players only as testimony.

**A few biological facts**

All evolved living species are sexual, because this mode of reproduction allows chromosomes to mix with each other at each generation and thus confers much greater adaptability to possible changes in the environment. Sex is determined at fecundation by the genetic lottery, which assigns the embryo two sex chromosomes forming its karyotype - the XX pair (female karyotype) or the XY pair (male karyotype) - at the same time as determining its uniqueness (we are all unique, all different). The karyotype directs the development of the phenotype, the set of anatomical, morphological and physiological characteristics of individuals.

During adolescence, the secretion of hormones, particularly testosterone, accentuates sexual differences. In males, skeletal and muscular development leads to inequalities in physical strength between men and women[191].
Women have narrower shoulders, lower average weight and lung capacity, smaller average height (by around 10 %) and lower haemoglobin levels. Their hearts are smaller (-15 % on average : 250 grams versus 300), their average heart rate is significantly higher, and their cardiac functions reach their maximum more quickly during exercise.

**Comparison of women's and men's world records**

This greater muscle development in men explains their superior sporting performance and the need to separate men and women in regional, national and international competitions. Girls and boys are equal in terms of sporting capacity before puberty. Beyond that, studies show that women are more enduring and more flexible, while men are faster and stronger. Female hormones promote joint and muscle laxity. This is especially true in the middle of the menstrual cycle or during pregnancy when oestrogen levels are highest. Strategy is said to be better developed in women who are less aggressive, more reflective and able to think before they act.
A comparison of men's and women's world records illustrates this, with men outperforming women by 10 % to 20 % in all disciplines except gymnastics and synchro-

---

191. Bassett A. J., Ahlmen A., Rosendorf J. M., Romeo A. A., Erickson B. J., Bishop M. E. "The Biology of Sex and Sport." *JBJS Rev.* 2020 Mar. ; 8(3):e0140. doi : 10.2106/JBJS.RVW.19.00140. PMID : 32224635.

nised swimming, known as artistic swimming, which are closer to dancing, where flexibility, agility and coordination are more important than muscular strength.
Here are a few examples of comparative world records (men/women): javelin throw (94 m/72 m), 50 m freestyle (46 s/51 s), 100 m sprint (9"58/10"49), shot put (23.37 m/22.63 m), 200 m race (19.19 s/21.34 s), 400 m race (43"03/47"60), weight lifting (488 kg/332 kg), marathon (42 km) (2 h 1 min 9 s/2 h 14 min 4 s), (1,500 m: 3 min 26/3 min 50), (5,000 m: 12 min 37 35/14 min 11 15), high jump (2 m 45/2 m 09), long jump (8.95 m/7 m 52). Note that in most sports, the quest for lightness (minimum weight) can be detrimental to power and therefore ultimately to results. The finalists at the world athletics championships in Budapest in August 2023 once again demonstrated this singularly in the sports disciplines of running and high jump. In tennis, Serena Williams admits that "she would lose 6-0, 6-0 in five minutes to Andy Murray".

These major differences in performance belie the gender ideology, which would have us believe that sex is a "social construct" that can be changed at will. They justify separating men and women in high-level sporting competitions[192].

192. Millard-Stafford M., Swanson A. E., Wittbrodt M. T. "Nature Versus Nurture: Have Performance Gaps Between Men and Women Reached an Asymptote?" *Int J Sports Physiol Perform.* 2018 Apr. 1; 13(4):530-535. doi: 10.1123/ijspp.2017-0866. Epub 2018 May 14. PMID: 29466055.

## Comparison of the physical capacities of trans women (born men) and cis women (born and remaining women)

Contrary to what trans activists[193][194][195] assert in the mainstream media, without citing any serious scientific study published by peer-reviewed medical journals, a man who claims to be a trans woman, even if he stuffs himself with oestrogen and has low testosterone levels, still retains broader shoulders, greater muscle mass, a greater respiratory capacity and a stronger heart, all of which make the competition with native-born women unfair [196][197][198][199][200].

---

193. https://www.slate.fr/story/232511/femmes-trans-ont-elles-avantage-competitions-sportives
194. https://toutesdesfemmes.fr/ressources/faq-sport-trans/
195. https://www.liberation.fr/sports/sportives-trans-lavantage-physique-cliche-sans-preuves-20230518_OXJ6QYJYWZBIFEES6SLHWDS66M/
196. Hilton E. N., Lundberg T. R. "Transgender Women in the Female Category of Sport: Perspectives on Testosterone Suppression and Performance Advantage." *Sports Med.* 2021 Feb.; 51(2):199-214. doi: 10.1007/s40279-020-01389-3. Erratum in: Sports Med. 2021 Oct; 51(10):2235. 503.
197. Knox T., Anderson L. C., Heather A. Transwomen in elite sport: scientific and ethical considerations. J Med Ethics. 2019 Jun; 45(6):395-403. doi: 10.1136/medethics-2018-105208. Epub 2019 Jun 19.
198. Hirschberg A. L., Elings Knutsson J., Helge T., Godhe M., Ekblom M., Bermon S., Ekblom B. "Effects of moderately increased testosterone concentration on physical performance in young women: a double blind, randomised, placebo controlled study." *Br J Sports Med.* 2020 May; 54(10):599-604. doi: 10.1136/bjsports-2018-100525. Epub 2019 Oct. 15. PMID: 31615775.
199. Alvares L. A. M., Santos M. R., Souza F. R., Santos L. M., Mendonça B. B., Costa E. M. F., Alves M. J. N. N., "Domenice S. Cardiopulmonary capacity and muscle strength in transgender women on long-term gender-affirming hormone therapy: a cross-sectional study." *Br J Sports Med.* 2022 Nov.; 56(22):1292-1298. doi: 10.1136/bjsports-2021-105400. Epub 2022 Oct. 4. Erratum in: *Br J Sports Med.* 2023 Feb.; 57(4):e2.
200. Senefeld J. W., Hunter S. K., Coleman D., Joyner M. J. "Case Studies in Physiology: Male to female transgender swimmer in college athletics." *J Appl Physiol* (1985). 2023 Apr. 1; 134(4):1032-1037. doi: 10.1152/japplphysiol.00751.2022. Epub 2023 Mar. 17. PMID: 36927141; PMCID: PMC10110692.

Dr Timothy Roberts, Associate Professor at the University of Missouri-Kansas City, found that trans women who had undergone hormone therapy for one year continued to outperform cisgender women, and although the gap narrowed after two years, trans women (hence men by birth) still ran 12 % faster than women (born women)[201]. L. A. Mr Alvares and his co-authors observed in 2022 that, even after more than ten years of hormone therapy, trans women's heart-lung capacity and strength exceed those of their cisgender counterparts[202], resulting in a de facto inequality that runs counter to the hopes of equality for all sought, and even affirmed, by the LGBTQ+ lobbies. Joanna Harper, a medical physicist at the British University of Loughborough and herself a transsexual athlete, admitted : "*Trans women are going to have strength advantages even after hormone therapy. I just don't see that as anything else but factual.*"[203]

In 2019, while the IOC[204] included trans women in high-level sporting competitions as long as they displayed

201. https://www.dw.com/en/fact-check-do-trans-athletes-have-an-advantage-in-elite-sport/a-58583988

202. A. Lam, S. Souza, Santos L. M., Mendonça B. B., Costa E. M. F., Alves M. J. N. N., Domenice S. "Cardiopulmonary capacity and muscle strength in transgender women on long-term gender-affirming hormone therapy : a cross-sectional study." *Br J Sports Med.* 2022 Nov. ; 56(22):1292-1298. doi : 10.1136/bjsports-2021-105400. Epub 2022 Oct. 4.

203. Harper J., O'Donnell E., Sorouri Khorashad B., McDermott H., Witcomb G. L. "How does hormone transition in transgender women change body composition, muscle strength and haemoglobin ? Systematic review with a focus on the implications for sport participation." *Br J Sports Med.* 2021 Aug. ; 55(15):865-872. doi : 10.1136/bjsports-2020-103106. Epub 2021 Mar. 1.

204. Comité international olympique.

low testosterone levels, T. Knox, L. C. Anderson and A. Bruyère concluded their study with the statement: "*The advantage given to transgender women by the IOC guidelines is an intolerable injustice.*"[205] A comparison of the recent results of women (born women) and men declared to be trans women amply confirms the physiological advantage retained by the latter in high-level competitions.

## A few examples of the unequal match between cis women (born women) and trans women

### In swimming

William Thomas was a mid-level swimmer who had never set a fast time in university competitions and was ranked 462nd when he competed as a man. After declaring himself a transgender woman, becoming Lia Thomas, he broke the University of Pennsylvania women's swimming record. And when women protested, he accused them of being transphobic, drawing more scathing remarks like those from Kentucky swimmer Riley Gaines, who tied with him in the women's 200m freestyle at the NCAA championships.

> "This take is selfish and shows utter disregard for women. Lia Thomas is not a brave, courageous woman who EARNED a national title. He is an arrogant cheat who STOLE a national title from a hardworking, deserving woman."

---

205. Knox T., Anderson L. C., Heather A., "Les femmes trans dans le sport d'élite: considérations scientifiques et éthiques." *Journal d'éthique médicale* 2019; 45: 395-403.

Caitlyn Jenner, a former transgender Olympic champion, described Lia Thomas' participation in a women's competition as "*one of the toughest, one of the hardest ... one of the worst things to happen to the trans community.*"[206] "*It just isn't fair, and we have to protect girl's sport in our schools.*"

**In cycling** too, men who identify themselves as trans women have easily racked up victories in women's competitions, often setting new records.

In New Zealand, a trans woman smashed the national women's mountain bike record at the championships in Wanaka. In Manchester (Great Britain), Rachel McKinnon broke the women's 35-39 world record at the Masters Track Cycling World Championships (2019).

In the USA, Austin Killips, who had never reached elite level before declaring herself trans and competing against women, took 3rd place in the Women Pro Race at the Really Rad Festival of Cyclocross and won the Verge Northampton International Cyclocross in Massachusetts.

Lesley Mumford, who declared his transition in 2017, won the 100-mile race in the 40-49 age category. But on the podium, he found himself alone, as the women he had beaten refused to stand next to a man.

Tiffany Thomas similarly dominated the cycling race in New York against her female rivals.

**In athletics,** high-level events have established the dominance of transgender women (born men) over competitors who were born and remain women.

206. https://www.breizh-info.com/2023/03/30/217643/les-trans-sexuels-enfin-interdits-dans-les-competitions-feminines-quelques-avancees/

The example of Halba Diouf, who, by "declaring" herself a woman, moved up from 980th place in the men's national rankings to 58th place in the women's world rankings, is a case in point.
South Africa's Caster Semenya, who was born a man, became a triple "women's" 800 m world champion after her transition. Between 2017 and 2020, two transgender women, hence born male, broke 17 women's records, depriving competitors who were born and remained female of 15 titles and 85 opportunities for sporting advancement.
Three of these women, Smith Selina Soule, Chelsea Mitchell and Ashley Nicoletti, felt they had been wronged by the rules of the Connecticut Interscholastic Athletic Conference and filed a complaint. The complaint was rejected at first instance, the judges finding that they were acting as "sore losers". The appeal is pending.

**In weightlifting as well**, the match between trans women and those born women is unfair : Anne Andres, a male weightlifter who identifies as a "woman", set a new women's national record at a championship in Brandon, Manitoba, beating the previous record by 95 kg.

**Allowing trans women to compete alongside sportswomen born female is contrary to feminism and sporting fairness**
As the 2024 Olympic Games draw nearer, the issue of transgender athletes taking part in women's competitions is becoming ever more pressing. Sixty years of feminist struggle risk resulting in the crowning of men draped in rainbow colours on podiums intended for women.

The International Olympic Committee has decided not to rule on this issue for the time being, leaving the international federations to conduct their own policies and establish their own rules for accepting or refusing trans athletes in competition.
The first competition, which already began in 2023, is the race for the greatest discrimination : those who are born female, with the physical capacities that nature has given them, against those who are born male and call themselves female, but have remained male by virtue of their sex, size, part of their musculature, heart and lungs, and in fact by virtue of their chromosomes. Neutral biologists keep explaining and repeating that you can't change sex. Manipulative propaganda cannot change reality, only deny it. The recent statement[207] from Sports Minister Amélie Oudéa-Castéra, when asked about the decision by the International Association of Athletics Federation (World Athletics), to exclude transgender people from women's competitions, is typical of the "on the fence attitude" dear to the French President : "*Not everyone is on that line. Scientific progress will inform the decision of these players*", adding : "*This is a difficult and evolving subject in which we have to navigate between two requirements, inclusion and respect for sporting fairness*". Including men by birth in women's sporting competitions because they say they are women and have undergone hormonal changes seriously undermines respect for gender equality, fairness and the rights of top-level sportswomen. Marguerite Stern, longstanding femi-

207. On the France Info channel.

nist activist[208], summed up the issue in an article in *Marianne*[209] and in *Le Figaro*[210] :

> "Under the guise of "combating discrimination", the various amendments concerning gender identity are a spit in the face of women, because if I understand their meaning correctly, they underlie the possibility that, on simple declaration, male individuals can take part in women's sporting competitions."
>
> "I'm not transphobic and I respect adults' sexual choices as long as they don't harm others, but there is no logical reason why women should be robbed of the titles they deserve in favour of a few men who don't shine in their birth category and who declare themselves uncomfortable in their birth body to compete against them. We can't accept these men stealing the podium from women who have worked hard to win the title."

Numerous scientific studies on the subject have convinced more and more sports federations of the validity of these remarks and have convinced them to prioritise equity for women over the inclusion of trans women born male.

In June 2022, the International Swimming Federation - now called World Aquatics - decided at an extraordinary

208. Still young, born in 1990, former member of FEMEN, initiator of the "Collages against Femicide" movement.

209. https://www.marianne.net/agora/tribunes-libres/reconnaitre-lidentite-de-genre-dans-une-competition-sportive-entre-en-contradiction-avec-le-fait-de-reconnaitre-le-sexe

210. https://www.lefigaro.fr/vox/societe/marguerite-stern-pourquoi-les-athletes-trans-n-ont-rien-a-faire-dans-les-competions-sportives-des-femmes-20230511

congress to set up an "open category" for transgender athletes. Each of us must always, within the limits of the principles of equity, guarantee the inclusion of all individuals regardless of their gender orientation, the Federation stated at the time. In practical terms, this decision[211] prohibits male-born athletes who declare themselves to be trans women from competing in the women's categories, unless they transitioned before puberty[212].

On 21 June 2022, the International Rugby League (IRL) announced[213] that transgender women will no longer be able to participate in women's rugby league matches until a consensual "full inclusion policy" has been established.

In June 2022, Sebastian Coe, President of the International Athletics Federation (World Athletics) said[214] :

> "My responsibility is to protect the integrity of women's sport… We have always believed, and repeated constantly, that biology trumps gender and we will continue to review our regulations in line with this."

---

211. International Swimming Federation (FINA). Eligibility policy for the men's and women's 2022 competition categories. https://resources.fina.org/fina/document/2023/03/27/dbc3381c-91e9-4ea4-a743-84c8b06debef/Policy-on-Eligibility-for-the-Men-s-and-Women-s-Competition-Categrories-Version-on-2023.03.24.pd

212. This does not, however, erase all the differences linked to chromosomes.

213. https ://www.intrl.sport/news/statement-on-transgender-particip-tion-in-women-s-international-rugby-league/

214. https://www.lefigaro.fr/sports/athletisme/athletisme-au-sujet-des-athletes-transgenres-sebastian-coe-la-biologie-l-emporte-sur-le-genre-20220621

On 23 March 2023, the International Athletics Federation (World Athletics) confirmed this choice in a press release[215]:

> "In regard to transgender athletes, the Council has agreed to exclude male-to-female transgender athletes who have been through male puberty from female World Rankings competition from 31 March 2023 … However, there are currently no transgender athletes competing internationally in athletics and consequently no athletics-specific evidence of the impact these athletes would have on the fairness of female competition in athletics. In these circumstances, the Council decided to prioritise fairness and the integrity of the female competition before inclusion."

On Friday 14 July 2023, the International Cycling Union announced that trans athletes will only be able to race with men. A decision aimed at "protecting the female category".

In August 2023, the International Chess Federation took the same decision. Is it a question of physical stamina during endless matches? The question remains to be clarified.

As doctors, we do not underestimate the suffering of transgender people, but we cannot accept that it should be used as an alibi for an unprecedented rollback of

215. https://www.francetvinfo.fr/sports/athletisme/sebastian-coe/athletisme-les-sportifs-transgenres-bannies-des-competitions-feminines_5728409.html

women's rights, which are already under threat throughout the world. We fully support the decisions taken by the international athletics, swimming, rugby and cycling federations, and it is highly likely that they will serve as models for the majority of federations in other sports once the subject has been studied objectively.
To enable trans athletes who wish to take part in high-level competitions without compromising fairness, it is certainly necessary to set up sports competitions that are "open" to all genders, enabling them to compare themselves with all the others[216] (comparable, incidentally, to mixed competitions), as proposed by the International Swimming Federation and the British Rowing and Cycling Federations. The competitors are perhaps mostly just sportsmen and women who want to win, and not necessarily obsessed with the visibility that trans activists put forward at every opportunity. Let's give them a fair chance, like everyone else.
Let sport triumph through open competition and let the best person win. Comparing records will also help to justify the logic of this decision.

---

216. Tidmas V., Halsted C., Cohen M., Bottoms L. "The Participation of Trans Women in Competitive Fencing and Implications on Fairness": *A Physiological Perspective Narrative Review. Sports (Basel).* 2023 Jul. 17; 11(7):133.

# 7.
# Teaching gender theory from nursery school to university

Sexuality education in schools is defined in the 2018 and 2023 circulars issued by the French Ministry of Education. The meaning of several terms used in the official circulars may be interpreted differently by different people. Since their personal understanding of the terms varies, the content taught in schools can sometimes be shocking.

In schools, sexuality education consists of three sessions each year from primary school upwards, and children are not allowed to opt out. The associations SOS Éducation and Les Mamans Louves have been compiling complaints from parents, such as the one on 31 January 2023 concerning a class of CM2 children (aged 10/11) who were forced to listen to a school nurse explain that: "*for pleasure a girl sucks the boy's penis*", "*the boy sucks the girl's vagina and can swallow something*", "*for pleasure the girl can gently fondle the boy's testicles*", "*you can have sex in the bottom*", "*you can change sex*"... "*take medicine to stop beard and hair growth*". They're only 10 years old!

These are just some of a number of complaints from parents[217].

This transformation of school into a hub of sex education has taken place surreptitiously, with the result that everyone started blaming their own school or their child's teacher, without ever imagining that the surreptitious change might be part of a widespread movement (until Pap Ndiaye's statement in 2022 that sexual education would be his priority), the September 2021 circular having gone unnoticed.

**2014 – The ABCD of equality**

Major transformations in French schools are nothing new. A decade has already elapsed since the Najat revolution and the "ABCD of equality". In late 2013, a 250-page report was officially aimed at "combating stereotypes", primarily in schools.[218] Commissioned by Najat Vallaud-Belkacem from the French public policy think tank Commissariat Général à la Stratégie, and coordinated by Marie-Cécile Naves and Vanessa Wisnia-Weill, the report entitled "Gender stereotypes and how to fight them: New Ideas from France", recommends influencing schools softly and subtly, in rather ambiguous terms, and contains no startling proposals. Its aims, however, were clearly denounced by Olivier Vial, spokesperson for the Observatoire de la Théorie du Genre:

217. «Quand l'éducation à la sexualité dérive et devient un danger pour la santé psychique de l'enfant »
https://actionetdemocratie.com/education-a-la-sexualite/
218. « La théorie du genre à petits pas à l'école » (lefigaro.fr)

> "It sounds a lot nicer than the Peillon-style dictates which sought to rely on the younger generations to create a change in people's mindset! It's simply the start of a soft propaganda effort to guide, through a series of insidious micro-incentives, people's behaviour and gradually replace one model of society with another."

Since 2014, the controversial ABCD of equality programmes have taken hold in schools. Meant to combat sexism, their introduction in 600 classes[219] has turned pupils into guinea pigs. This *experiment* on pupils was supported jointly by the French Education Minister Vincent Peillon and his fellow Minister for Women's Rights Najat Vallaud-Belkacem. A total of ten volunteer *Académies*, i.e. French regional education authorities, involving more than 600 classes, were enlisted into the programme, designed to "deconstruct gender stereotypes" and "*foster a culture of equality and respect between girls and boys from the earliest age, by addressing the attitudes of those working in education and the prejudices of pupils*". The stated aim is to "*raise awareness among pupils of the ways in which girls and boys are represented and assigned roles, thereby influencing career choices that are known to be gendered*". However, it is a "*more comprehensive approach aimed at influencing attitudes that also encompasses schools*". Olivier Vial, president of UNI, France's Inter-University Union, called for vigilance, as did leaders of the *Association des Familles Catholiques*, who feared that schools would undermine the values passed on by parents.

In 2014, several thousand pupils, from nursery to Year 5, were introduced to this concept of "equality" through

219. « École : un nouveau genre de programme » (lefigaro.fr)

teaching sessions delivered by teachers. Examples of teaching sessions were the "aesthetic representations of children, women and men" over the centuries, from Rigaud's portrait of Louis XIV wearing high heels to Yves Saint Laurent's dinner jacket for women in 1966, and reflections on "the figure of female beauty" in fairy tales. The stated aim was to show children that notions of masculine and feminine change with society and time.
For the two ministries, the official aim was to "*raise awareness among pupils of the ways in which girls and boys are represented and assigned roles, and to help teachers in this task by offering guidance within existing official curricula : science, physical education and sport, language skills, history, and so forth*"[220]. Teachers were however given a degree of freedom in their classrooms. The message was fairly gentle, confined in some cases to a judicious attack on certain preconceived ideas by pointing out, for example, that girls are just as capable of pursuing higher scientific studies as boys.

It was in 2014 that the first attempt was made to stop the damage being done within the French education system, in reaction to the movement known coyly as the "*ABCD of equality*", which led to the intrusion into state schools of discourse that had no business being there. This initial reaction by parents was caricatured by the press in almost univocal terms as "*rumour launched and propagated by militants close to the extreme right*", used by

220. *Ibid.*, 11.

France Info[221], RTL[222], *Le Figaro*[223], and *Le Journal du dimanche*[224]. An attempt at resistance appeared in the media via the website of the movement "JRE2014", "*an unprecedented national action to save our children*", explained the leaflet, urging parents to give the following reason for their child's absence the following day: "*day of withdrawal from school to ban gender theory in all schools*". "*National Education Minister Vincent Peillon, following in the footsteps of his predecessor Luc Chatel, wants to extend and make official the teaching of gender theory [...] at the start of the 2014 school year [...] Hundreds of schoolchildren have already fallen victim to these trial programmes,*" the text added, referring to the ABCD of equality. "*Already, activists from the LGBT (lesbian, gay, bisexual and transgender) lobby are inviting themselves into the classroom*", the leaflet explained, going on to say that "*Our children's education belongs to us*" and calling for the return of "*a Ministry of Public Instruction*".

What appears more openly now than in 2014 is the early sexualisation of children. The harmful and authoritarian role of the WHO, which is supposed to be concerned with health and not education, is increasingly apparent as the Organisation is trying to impose its

221. https://www.francetvinfo.fr/societe/education/l-etrange-rumeur-sur-la-theorie-du-genre-a-l-ecole_1680537.html

222. https://www.rtl.fr/actu/theorie-du-genre-une-rumeur-totalement-mensongere-7769254407

223. Théorie du genre: des élèves absents du fait d'une étrange rumeur (lefigaro.fr) https://fr.search.yahoo.com/search?fr=mcafee&type=E210FR0G0&p=Th%C3%A9orie+du+genre+%3A+des+%C3 %A91 %C3 %A8ves+absents+du+-fait+d %27une+%C3 %A9trange+rumeur+(lefigaro.fr)

224. https://www.lejdd.fr/Societe/Des-eleves-absents-du-fait-d-une-folle-rumeur-650617-3190055

hegemony over all countries and turn itself into a world government.

> "The main change in these sex education sessions is that they introduce the notion of pleasure and start from the premise that the child "must become aware that sexuality is an integral part of being a healthy human being". [...] These sessions are based on the Standards for Sexuality Education in Europe (published in 2014), a document presented as a WHO 'framework for policy makers, educational and health authorities and specialists."[225]

How can certain principles of this framework cause considerable psychological damage in children[226]?

Page 38 of the Standards for Sexuality Education in Europe[227] explains, in the matrix, that it is necessary to:

> "inform children aged 0 to 4 about enjoyment and pleasure when touching one's own body, early childhood masturbation, that children aged 0 to 4 should be allowed to express their own needs, wishes and boundaries, for example in the context of "playing doctor" (p: 38), by helping them to develop a "curiosity regarding their own body and others' bodies".

---

225. « Quand l'éducation à la sexualité dérive et devient un danger pour la santé psychique de l'enfant. »
https://actionetdemocratie.com/education-a-la-sexualite/
226. *Nouveau Monde* — « Conférence Dr Nicole Delépine: STOP au sabotage de l'école et à la sexualisation de l'enseignement » (nouveau-monde.ca)
227. *Nouveau Monde* — « L'OMS et ses standards dépravés pour l'éducation sexuelle en Europe » (nouveau-monde.ca)

Any sane person will be surprised by the "0 years", but the WHO explains that sexual education begins at birth and that "babies touch themselves and sometimes their genitals" (p. 13)[228].

As far as children aged 4 to 6 are concerned, it is explained that:

> They should be informed of "sexual feelings (closeness, enjoyment, excitement) as a part of all human feelings", and that if the experience or feeling is not good, you do not always have to comply".

Ages 9 to 12:

> to be informed about "pleasure, masturbation, orgasm", "the differences between gender identity and biological sex" [and enable them to] "*make a conscious decision to have sexual experiences or not*"; [to develop] "*the understanding of sexuality as a learning process*" (p. 44) and "*take responsibility in relation to safe and pleasant sexual experiences for oneself and others*".

For adolescents aged 12 to 15, the WHO recommends information on "*how to enjoy sexuality in an appropriate way*" (p. 47).

The article by Action & Démocratie rightly questions the scientific basis of such guidance and the authors' actual knowledge of children's psychosexual development, guid-

228. *Ibid.*, 236.

ance that they wish to impose on everyone dependent on the WHO by means of enforceable treaties as of 2024. It is time for Westerners to wake up and reject these unacceptable agreements, which have already been rejected by a great many countries.

> "Although children are sexed, they are not sexualised in the adult sense. For their psychological well-being, it is important to respect their modesty, intimacy and sexual immaturity. Adults have a duty to protect children and teach them to protect themselves from predators, but under no circumstances should adults introduce children to adult sexuality."

**2021 - The Blanquer circular**

The ABCD of Equality in 2014 was an initial foray – the minister at the time denying the existence of a gender theory, let alone its teaching in schools despite the evidence to the contrary – that ushered in the introduction to schools of the Blanquer circular in September 2021[229]. The circular imposed attitudes on teachers, staff and pupils and yet was not discussed or highlighted in the mainstream media.

> "From nursery school through to secondary school, schools are being asked to take steps to listen to, support and protect "children who are transgender or who have questions about their gender identity".

229. The signed circular by Jean-Michel Blanquer", appeared in the *Bulletin officiel* of 30 September 2021.

Trans activists want to make their struggle the standard-bearer of progressive struggles in the 21st century and have long been putting pressure on the French education system to make the protection and promotion of trans-identity a priority. They have won the day and have now infiltrated all decision-making circles, ministries, large companies and government departments, where their numbers are very high compared with the percentage of this small minority (0.1 %) of the population. This was borne out in schools by the statements made by Minister Pap Ndiaye in September 2022.

**Examples of injunctions given to the teachers, carers, administrators and parents who work with children and adolescents**

- ***Recognise a "preferred name"*** where it differs from the birth name. Pupils are free to choose a new name and the administration and teaching staff must take this on board as soon as the young person's wish is expressed (including within 48 hours from Friday to Monday). However, civil status alone is recognised when it comes to national examinations. A simple circular cannot override civil law.

- ***Respect changes of pronouns***. For example, when a male pupil wishes to be called "she" (or a female pupil wishes to be called "he"), teaching staff and other pupils must agree to this and apply it (including other young pupils who find it very difficult to understand and therefore to follow). The sensitivities of the other pupils are dismissed.

**- *Ensure "respect for choices in matters of dress and appearance", "without gender-specific requirements".*** There is no reason to stigmatise make-up, skirts and heels for transgender girls, if they are accepted for girls who are born "cisgender" in the neo-vocabulary of transsexuals. (Note that the current controversy over the abaya, which was settled by the new minister in August 2023, is leading many to call for a uniform for all – or at least identical, simple, neutral clothing for all. This might also solve the problem of high heels and make-up, which have no place in schools).

**- *Provide mixed-sex toilets*.** This provision must also be respected on school outings. And, of course, in boarding schools. This leads to huge problems, as we shall see later.

According to the circular, teachers have a "*duty to support young people and show them the greatest possible understanding, and allow them to explore different paths without stigmatising them*". When dealing with students who are questioning their gender identity, "*we need to be attentive to their needs and their specific experiences and reassure them that they have the right to ask questions*".
And what about the other pupils who do not understand what is happening to their classmate and in turn are distressed?
A child comes out as transgender in a class and then all the other children are left perplexed in front of a teacher who has no freedom to reassure them or help them understand this new policy, in which the biology that knows only two sexes is denied. Imagine the teaching skills, the

degree of tolerance, kindness, empathy, intellectual and emotional intelligence that teachers must develop to safeguard the wellbeing of the children entrusted to them in this scenario!
This insistence on the respect due to transgender pupils rules out "*questioning the questioning*". Should a child with a faltering sense of self who is "searching" for his or her identity necessarily be guided (proselytising organisations are increasingly prominent on social networks) towards a new gender identity?

How could this circular have passed without arousing indignation and a call to common sense among both teachers and parents in September 2021, and what enormous responsibility have the mainstream media and journalists assumed for keeping quiet about its publication, highly symbolic of the loss of freedom of expression, freedom of thought and, ultimately, freedom to teach?
How could we suddenly accept the ban on talking to children and very young teenagers about their natural and universal unease surrounding the transformation of their bodies, about what puberty means not only for their physical appearance, but also for the intellectual and emotional feelings linked to their hormonal changes?
Have we returned to the Middle Ages? Even then, weren't mothers and grandmothers closer to children and able to teach them the "fifty shades" of metamorphosis from caterpillar to butterfly, from child to a woman who would soon to be tasked by nature with the perpetuation of the species, from a little boy to a man whose more developed musculature assigns him the role of protector?

Why deny the illnesses that sometimes go hand in hand with puberty, that have always existed, from depression to autism or eating disorders, from anorexia to bulimia, and so forth? In the absence of psychiatrists (on the verge of extinction as a result of the destruction of the health-care system over the past forty years) able to diagnose and treat those who have difficulty getting through this period (followed swiftly by their friends, through group contagion), should we be handing children over to the social network influencers who turn these conditions, all of which can be remedied with appropriate care, into gender identity disorders?
It seems that young people with autistic symptoms are over-represented among prospective transitioners. Is this by chance or the result of social networking?

And schools are expected to accept this totalitarian dictate! Who voted for this?
Under the pretext of "respecting the dignity of pupils", teachers are being judged according to the way they support transgender pupils. But how much leeway will they have to criticise, challenge or question such a desire in a child, and more importantly help him or her discover his or her real concerns or indeed, at times, obsessions that overshadow everything else (at the sight of a pimple or unexpected hair)? None at all!

The circular specifies that these measures will only apply if the pupil has the consent of both parents. How then does one object to a "private", family decision? Because objecting would be considered an act of "transphobia".

Bear in mind that seemingly consenting parents can still be threatened with accusations of ill-treatment if they refuse the child's demands (or even threatened with having custody of their child removed by the family courts if they do not acquiesce). What's more, help from professional psychiatrists or psychologists has been less forthcoming in recent years because those advocating caution are often accused of transphobia too.

School authorities, obsessed with their famous "*don't rock the boat*" policy, want no accusations of Islamophobia[230], and now transphobia, levelled against them. "*Teachers are advised not to broach controversial issues too directly (secularism, freedom of expression, the Islamist mass shooting at the offices of Charlie Hebdo, teaching about the Holocaust, etc.), so as not to open up a new front with the progressive camp*".

Worse still, should it be up to teachers to act as intermediaries in establishing a dialogue, "supporting" and helping young people faced with recalcitrant parents? What has any of this got to do with schools, especially when it comes to freedom to act?

In *La Question trans* (Le débat/Gallimard), Claude Habib describes the unease, indeed inability, of adults to deal composedly with a child's or adolescent's request to "change their body".

> "Parents are afraid of being abusive, of not responding favourably to their child's suffering. They may be intimi-

230. Think of the many controversies that have led to the refusal to name certain secondary schools after Samuel Paty, the teacher murdered by Islamists for defending free speech.

> dated by psychiatrists who have no hesitation in making them feel guilty: "If your child commits suicide because he is in the wrong body, responsibility will lie with you".[231]

**Validation by the Conseil d'État**

The Ministry of Education's circular was challenged by one parent, who referred the matter to the Conseil d'État, citing the law that stipulates: "*No citizen may bear a surname or forename other than those stated in his birth certificate*". In a decision handed down on Wednesday 28 September 2022, the Conseil refused to overturn the section of the circular whereby transgender pupils were allowed to use the name of their choice at school.

The Conseil d'État ruled that the use of a different first name by pupils was an "internal school matter" and stated that only in national qualification examinations should the first name recorded in the civil status register be used.

Children, who are deemed legally incapable, are given the power to coerce adults as soon as they talk about gender. Nevertheless, naming remains a major anthropological invariant.

Giving children the power to erase all trace of filiation conferred by their parents and impose a new first name makes them self-made men, the embodiment of the absolute individualism advocated by managerial ideology. The message is clear: feelings are the law, or rather tran-

231. Cf. the chapter on trans suicides, which clearly shows that suffering, unfortunately, does not improve with the multiple "aggressions" of medical and surgical treatments.

scend the law. This interference by schools in pupils' private lives is bound to give rise to conflict[232].

When dissidents are famous, these objections come to the fore in tweets such as Booba's: "*If my son comes home from school one day and tells me his name is Mireille, we will have a serious problem.*" On 30 September 2022, Caroline de Haass replied to Booba: "*Transphobia kills, delete*" and on 1 October 2022, Booba replied: "*If anyone comes up to my 7-year-old son and tells him he can be called Jacqueline and have his willy cut off, I'll take him on a tour of Mars and its suburbs. Keep it up!*"

In the USA, clashes of opinion between woke schools and parents are leading to tragedies[233].

Here is an instructive example of one mother's struggle:

> No white knight would be riding in to rescue their kids—they were it. California mom Erin Friday, 56, found out she was it for her then 11-year-old daughter. It started innocently enough: just a few boyish-sounding nicknames and a couple of extra letters from the alphabet. But innocent it was not.
>
> A few girls, including Friday's young one, were heard chattering in the front yard about some new things they learned at school. They were hip to fresh trends while, in their minds, boring old mom was the know-nothing dinosaur who was way behind the times.

---

232. https://www.fdesouche.com/2022/10/01/prise-de-bec-entre-la-militante-caroline-de-hass-et-le-rappeur-booba-apres-un-tweet-juge-transphobe/

233. Courtesy of Erin Friday USA, "California Mom Reclaims Young Daughter from Clutches of Trans Agenda in Middle School – Here's How.", by Michael Wing, 28 May 2023, *The Epoch Times*.

"Five girls, each one of them picked a label that was on the alphabet, and they actually kind of giggled at me and said, 'You're cis, and you don't understand,'" explained Mrs Friday. "I had never heard the term "cis" before, and then they said, "OK, boomer.".

It was 2019, and Friday's daughter was in seventh grade. This was the mom's first eye-opening moment: "What the heck are they teaching our kids at school?!" she wondered. Curiosity turned to concern as this gender-fixated culture germinated. "Oh, it's probably just puberty," she thought at first.

Friday's once-girly daughter—a huge "My Little Pony" fan—started draping herself in baggy sweatshirts. Friday thought it just "an act of shyness" with the blooming of womanhood; Friday had experienced as much. But as the "My Little Pony" fan crossed into "soldier girl" territory, lacing up combat boots; as long-haired female friends started assuming guys' names; as the purple and green hair dye broke out, mom's worry worsened.

*A poison seed in middle school sex education*

It became cool to have a label. As one girl identified as pansexual, another called herself polyamorous (open to multiple partners), nonsensically. "Half her Girl Scout troupe came out as transgender," Friday said. Out came the breast binders. Girly voices suspiciously dropped low overnight.

"My daughter picked 'pansexual.' She was 11. There's nothing sexual about my 11-year-old daughter," Friday said. "A couple picked 'lesbian,' but nobody picked 'straight'.

"Whatever your teacher says is gold and truthful," Friday said. "The two most important people in a child's life are the parents and then the teacher." She had trusted them, and the school had let her down.

A third-party group came in and taught five hours of sex ed. With a name like Health-Connected, it sounds innocuous, though they are anything but.

"They spent an entire hour of the five hours of instruction teaching about gender ideology, having the 'genderbread man' cartoon—where they point to the brain and they point to the body parts—and they essentially say that you can have a female brain and a male body, or vice versa."

It was for fear of the students who came out as their "authentic self" that teachers kowtowed and treated them differently, Friday said. They were lauded as amazing and special, regarded as unicorns, and elevated to the status of superstar. "Kids who are sort of on the fringes, without a lot of big friend groups, or maybe a little weird, come out as trans and hit stardom," she said. "If you're white, middle class or affluent, and straight, you're an oppressor, you're boring, there's nothing special about you."

There is no freedom for parents threatened by the juvenile court if they are not sufficiently cooperative[234]. The school interferes in the child's life without informing the parents. What would you have done?

Over time, this unwholesome fruit ripened. In 2020 when COVID saw students locked down and learning from home, Friday was shocked to learn the public high school had been using her daughter's male pronoun and

234. As in France, parents who refuse a clinical trial for their child, or even a simple DTP vaccine, can be prosecuted.

> confronted the administration. In a phone call, they told her the reason for this was to provide a "safe space," which Friday found ludicrous. Her daughter was just down the hall from her.
> "They responded back very, very strangely [about the matter of changing her name], 'Oh, well, we didn't do it legally,'" Friday said. "I told them, 'You can't actually, I'm the parent. Remember that. I am the parent. You are not the parent.'

The college dared to inform social services.

> "I guess I must be 'unsafe' because I use her female name, and her female pronouns. And then Child Protective Services [CPS] showed up at my door. The police came later."
> CPS deemed her daughter a suicide risk, citing a search she did on her school iPad. Though CPS ended up dropping its investigation, Friday was infuriated by the school's using a suicide fear as a guise for a possible abuse claim for her confronting their brazen secret social transition of her daughter.

This loving and intelligent mother helped her to understand what was going on, particularly in this delirious period of "plandemics" and family isolation that has led so many young people to fail at school, become depressed or even commit suicide. Need we remind readers of the wealth of medical literature on the psychological disorders suffered by children and adolescents as a result of school closures and physical isolation from their friends? This worldwide experiment has at least shown that digital-everything is just an illusion.

Mrs Friday understood that her daughter's lockdown-induced depression had more to do with her gender outburst than anything else. She wasn't the only child sent spiralling into a mental tailspin by COVID. It was clear as day. However, the medical establishment has been thoroughly manipulated.

> [...] The therapist insisted Friday's memory of her daughter's girliness was "incorrect". [...] "I have a son, they're very different." The therapist flaunted the "41 % chance of committing suicide" trope before Mrs Friday. "When I queried her about the study, it was very clear to me that she didn't read it. I had," Friday said. "I would have been fired from my job as a lawyer if I ever cited a case that I didn't read. So that's what the therapist who failed to treat her daughter's depression got. Fired.

To Mrs Friday, it seemed the whole world had gone mad. The battle to reclaim her daughter and start some "deprogramming" with her was a long journey from which many parents would do well to draw inspiration. We'll return to this later.

**Rehabilitation of the role of parents in England**

Things, nonetheless, are changing, particularly in Anglo-Saxon countries. In England, teachers will now have to tell parents if their child is questioning his or her gender identity[235].

On Monday 17 July 2023, UK Minister for Education Kemi Badenoch announced the forthcoming publication

235. Supplied by Madmoizelle.

of a raft of guidelines limiting transsexual propaganda in schools. Speaking on the BBC, she said that teachers would be given new guidance to better manage cases of "*gender distress*". The guidance was accused by pro-trans journalists of *flouting the pupil's consent and ignoring the child's potentially hostile family environment, even if it means putting the child in danger*!

**"Ensuring parents know what is going on with their children at school".**

According to the new guidelines, teachers will now be obliged to inform parents if their child is questioning his or her gender identity. According to the Minister, the aim of this measure is to "*ensure parents know what is going on at school.*"

As our Guardian colleagues report, the new guidance requires teachers to always consult parents if a child wishes to be called by another name or wear a different uniform. Schools are also advised not to use a child's preferred pronoun until parents give their consent. Finally, the guidance advises teachers that any pupil who wants to self-identify as a different gender should first undergo a period of reflection.

**Shows imposed on schools**

Interference in schools is not limited to "teaching" sessions conducted by campaigning groups who promote gender theory. School outings are now being organised, and families have discovered just how frequent and manipulative they are.

For instance, the Département of Ille-et-Vilaine and the

Region of Brittany subsidised a school outing for children from the Jean-Rostand school in Rennes to attend a show[236] promoting gender theory and sex change on 20 March 2023. Reports of school trips to the theatre to see NORMALITO have been passed on to associations combating wokeism in schools.
Here are the comments made by Year 5 children to their parents after the show:

> "What's depressive? The boy was depressed and violent."
> "He's my age and he ran away!", "Is it normal to run away when you're little? Isn't it dangerous?"
> "It's not right to *be normal*!
> "What's a zebra girl?
> "The man wasn't born in the right body, so he dresses like a woman."

In the brochure for the show (funded by the DRAC, the French Regional Directorate of Cultural Affairs), there are many shocking elements. "*Normal is not normal*", "*It's normal to feel better in the home of other parents than in your own*", "*The pee lady who was born in the wrong body...*"
While it is normal to respect the informed sexual choices of adults, this misleading transsexual propaganda aimed at children must be firmly condemned as it risks psychologically disturbing them at a difficult age. It needlessly rekindles discord in society and harms sexual minorities,

236. « Camille, une fille dans un corps de garçon, une fille qui attend la mutation. » English translation: Camille, a girl in a boy's body, awaiting change.

just as previous campaigns featuring gays and trans people have been followed by an increase in incidents against these minorities.

**Academic consequences**

While the fanatics who truly believe that children can change sex are very much in the minority, professionals in education, psychotherapy and medicine who remain silent are complicit in this contemporary scandal.

Since the 1980s, this theory has gradually and insidiously invaded state school education - which is now more obsessed with teaching young people about diverse sexualities and notions of gender - masculine, feminine, non-binary, neutral, trans, fluid or other - than with reading, writing and arithmetic.

University teaching has been transformed by the exclusion of dissenting voices (or those merely open to discussion), who have been banned from lectures at Paris's Sciences Po, Grenoble and Clermont-Ferrand universities, among others. As both the victim and the author of mass manipulation, it has lost its role in emancipating the masses and has become a silo, a sector devoid of all intellectual richness[237].

**Sexualisation in schools[238]**

Since the arrival of Minister Pap Ndiaye at the Ministry of National Education in September 2022 (until July 2023), the government's desire to apply WHO guidelines on sex

237. *Nouveau Monde* — Interview with Prof. Mattias DESMET on mass conditioning (nouveau-monde.ca)

238. « Sexualisation des enfants à l'école » (odysee.com)

education, as set out on its website, according to age group, from birth onwards, has been plain to see. Many countries around the world are, however, fighting back.

A highly successful piece of propaganda in the USA is the US Gender Queer book, which contains depictions of oral sex, masturbation and homosexual acts, and can easily be found in the libraries of some American primary schools. Maia Kobabe, "non-binary" author of the controversial book, sees nothing wrong with the book and says that all these things are "part of life".

A video of an Illinois librarian recommending the publication shocked those who had never heard of the book. Some called it "*distributing pornography to minors*", while others said the librarian should be arrested[239]. "*Some babies know they are transgender from the womb*", according to Harvard psychologist Kerry McGregor. In a video published and since deleted, McGregor argued that babies should be able to decide their sex, even though their brains are not fully developed. "*A good portion of children do know as early as seemingly from the womb and they will usually express their gender identity as very young children – some as soon as they can talk*", says Ms McGregor in the video[240], before admitting that her clinic takes in children "*all the way down to ages 2 and 3 and usually up to age of 9*", and explaining to parents how to best "*support*" their supposedly "different" child by making sure that the child has the space and support to explore their gender[241].

239. https://t.me/akounamatatatv [Video]
240. Harvard Children's Hospital: Babies Know in the Womb if They're Transgender: Grabien News
241. https://www.anguillesousroche.com/etats-unis/un-hopital-americain-declare-que-les-bebes-savent-quils-sont-transgenres-des-leur-naissance/ t.me/StreetReporters1

Sexual identity is determined for life at fertilisation by the pairing of the sex chromosomes; gender is merely a feeling, a social appearance that should be respected in adults (while honestly informing them of the medical and surgical consequences of their choice to undergo medical transition), but not promoted in minors whose physical, emotional and mental development is not yet complete (not before the age of 25 for the brain).

In conclusion, it is vital to inform children for their protection, provided that we respect their maturity, modesty and sensitivity. The aim is to respond fully to their questions on an individual basis, without getting ahead of them.
Intimate matters cannot be tackled in public.

# 8
# The detransitioners: disappointments with sex reassignment and accounts of "detransitioning"

**"Propaganda destroyed my life"**

Lobbies, fashion, business, the Internet, associations invited by the French Minister of Education to talk about sex education in schools, misleading and/or ideological advertising, whether sincere or motivated by huge profits at all levels, along with cinema, television (whose subsidies depend on their compliance with the accepted orthodoxy), and attention-grabbing social networks[242] all feed into the conviction of many teenagers who "*feel uncomfortable in their skin*" that their worries (which are entirely "normal" at this stage of life) reflect a mistaken "gender".

242. Some of these influencers are also paid by the lobbies, as seen with the Covid tests and injections which they advertised - often they themselves convinced and manipulated - to millions of young people who followed them, some of whom dying from complications of the pseudo-vaccine. Others, now disabled, post their stories on the Internet.

When they consult specialists in gender dysphoria, having swiftly been referred to “the experts” by their GPs or psychologists who feel out of their depth, they often find themselves facing ideological transgender activists and/or those interested in lucrative business opportunities, who would have them believe that a sex change would solve their problem. These doctors quickly prescribe hormone treatments, followed by surgery, without always informing them objectively of the possible complications of the treatments, the irreversible nature of the surgery, and the outcomes, which often fall short of expectations.

After a few years, a growing number of transsexuals realise that their discomfort persists or has increased as a result of disappointment with the outcome of the transition. They are no happier and sometimes their distress has even increased, hence the terrible suicide figure of 40 % (see dedicated chapter). They reidentify with their birth sex[243] and try to revert. These people are called detransitioners[244]. This is a taboo subject in the media and among researchers, and for this reason it is difficult to quantify[245], but testimonials from detransitioners or people tempted to detransition are multiplying[246].

243. https://www.observatoirepetitesirene.org/post/d%C3%A9transition-ils-ont-chang%C3%A9-de-sexe-et-ils-regrettent

244. https://files.cargocollective.com/c523136/01_Post-Trans_Booklet_FR.pdf

245. Detransitioners say that they are no longer under the care of their medical team if they wish to revert, and are therefore counted in the statistics as “lost to follow-up” and not as disappointed.

246. See on Telegram : “detransition support group”.

## Some testimonials on the Internet

Oli London, a British influencer with over a million followers on TikTok, recounts his transition[247] and the dozens of operations he underwent. The transition cost him more than $271,000 and was followed by a desire to detransition[248]. Quite quickly, just months after starting his transition journey, he questioned his way of thinking, asked himself why he had put himself through all this, and whether he was happy. Gradually, the starkest reality dawned on him : he was still profoundly unhappy despite his transition.

Steven A. Richards[249] provides us with another testimony.

> "I became a male-to-female transsexual when I was only 15 years old. Bullying at school, instability at home, and a lack of close friends had left me looking for somewhere to belong, and the transgender movement happily provided one — at the cost of my health and sanity. Living as a transgender woman left me delusional, paranoid, and sick. Despite this, I stayed transgender for eight years. The nature of the transgender movement makes it almost impossible to escape and pushes the people within it to adopt radical beliefs and irreversibly harm themselves.
>
> Coming to terms with what I lost has been the hardest thing I've ever done. Deciding to de-transition cost me

---

247. https://www.valeursactuelles.com/clubvaleurs/societe/entretien-oli-london-confession-dun-trans-repenti?uid=ODAyNDQy
248. https://www.breizh-info.com/2023/02/25/215950/devenir-trans-puis-regretter-le-temoignage-de-oli-london/
249. https://religion-is-a-mental-illness.tumblr.com/post/695974373122850816/embed

> many close friends and forced me to rebuild my whole life. For some members of the movement — those who have lost ties with their family, who rely on the community for food and housing — de-transitioning isn't an option. Many of them still live in the miserable world I escaped from, hoping that the next step in their transition — a new name, a new set of pronouns, another year of hormones, another surgery — will bring them the happiness they were promised. But, as I learned, it never can."

This testimony is particularly poignant, and makes us feel ashamed and pained as doctors, because clearly this man and all the former friends he is talking about were not properly advised by the medical profession, due either to incompetence or self-interest[250]. Our Hippocratic oath, the key phrase of which is "above all do no harm", has been flouted, as happened on a massive scale by the vast majority of doctors during the Covid crisis, and is still happening today.

Chris Beck, a former US Navy Special Forces soldier, described his change of sex as follows[251]. "*I was used ... I was very naive, I was in a really bad way, and I got taken advantage of. I got propagandized*", denouncing "*propaganda*" as having "*destroyed my life*".

Mikael Kruse, a 36-year-old Swede, had a sex change in his late twenties, but it never resolved his discomfort,

250. This little book is an attempt to "make amends" to these people in the name of our corporate mistreatment of them.
251. https://nypost.com/2022/12/11/retired-navy-seal-chris-beck-who-came-out-as-trans-announces-detransition-destroyed-my-life/

and after seven years he finally detransitioned. "*I think it's good to take a break to understand what's going on*", he told AFP[252]. A new diagnosis revealed he had Asperger's Syndrome as well as Attention Deficit Disorder, and the suffering he thought was related to his gender was due to other factors.

Ash Eskridge, a student in Missoula, Montana (USA), began transitioning into a boy at the age of 13. She said she felt depressed at the age of 12 and had been manipulated by social media influencers into believing she was transgender.

Ash made a social transition, which involved changing her name, wardrobe and cutting her hair. At the age of 16, Ash started taking testosterone and her voice became deeper. She realised she had made a mistake in April 2023, after feeling "unnatural" with body hair and a deep voice, and began to detransition. Today, the mother-daughter duo is speaking out and pleading for better mental health care for teenagers in situations similar to Ash's.

Aleksa Lundberg, long considered a kind of ambassador for the trans community in Sweden, also regrets her transition[253], and in particular her sterilisation[254]. When she began the intensive process of changing from male

252. https://www.france24.com/en/live-news/20230208-sweden-puts-brakes-on-treatments-for-trans-minors
253. https://www.deutschlandfunkkultur.de/zweifel-einer-transfrau-man-wird-schnell-transphob-genannt-100.html
254. https://www.huffpost.com/entry/transgender-forced-sterilization_n_1071328

to female at the age of 17, Lundberg hadn't given much thought to the fact that she would have to be sterilised.

> "I believed I had to give up every vestige of being male to complete the process. I cried and shouted for joy when that final piece of paper dropped in the mailbox telling me that I was now legally a woman."

When she woke up and realised that she had lost an important part of her sexual sense, it was a real shock for her. She realised that she was in fact a gay feminine man who felt she had to change her body to be accepted.

Something else became clear to her : young people base their decision for or against treatment on the sunny stories that trans people tell in the media. But they hide an important part of their true story.

Elie, a 24-year-old Belgian social sciences student, started taking testosterone at the age of 16, followed by a mastectomy at 17 and a detransitioning process at 20. She is now dedicated to working harder to improve the lives of dysphoric people and women and girls who believe they are gender non-conforming.

Nele is a 27-year-old freelance illustrator and graphic designer from Germany. She began her transition at the age of 20, only to end it after two years of testosterone and a mastectomy[255]. She recently published a comic strip on the theme of detransitioning.

255. "Hello, we are Elie and Nele" https://post-trans.com/About-Us

**The judicialisation of gender politics: negligence, disinformation and abuse**

Kayla Lovdahl, an 18-year-old Californian, is suing her former doctors and two hospitals, accusing them of negligence for performing a double mastectomy on her at the age of 13, when she needed attention and psychotherapy and not cross-sex hormones or mutilating surgery.

She says that she was "*exposed to online transgender influencers who prompted her to erroneously believe she was transgender when she was 11*" and that after a single 75-minute transition evaluation, doctors put her on puberty blockers and testosterone at the age of 12, before performing a double mastectomy six months later. At the age of 17, Lovdahl realised that she was not trans and began to detransition. Neglect, abuse…

Sinead was 29 in 2020. A series of painful and difficult experiences in her youth led her to reject femininity and desire to be a man. Now she understands that "transitioning" hasn't solved her problems and concerns, and is reverting to her birth gender.

At the age of 16, Jannika Häggström's youngest daughter told her mother that she was a man. The mother refused to consent to sex reassignment treatment. At the age of 18, the adult daughter had her breasts amputated and took testosterone. At the age of 20, just two years later, she realised that it was all an obsessive fixation.

Walt Heyer describes his painful journey[256]: sexual abuse as a child followed by depression, feelings of depersonalisation and rejection of his own gender as an adult male. He states that too often, post-traumatic stress symptoms related to sexual violence are interpreted as gender dysphoria with sex reassignment as the solution.

Charlie Evans, a British science journalist who was born a woman, lived as a man for ten years before realising that transitioning was a cop-out, not a solution to her worries, and living as a woman again.
She warns against making decisions too early, too quickly and without sufficient discussion.

> "I knew I was a boy because I liked cars and trucks and mud and boxing and girls. I knew I was a boy because I didn't act like a girl. Nothing about my character felt 'girly' and trans ideology says everyone feels like their gender. I didn't feel like a girl. I knew I was a boy because I meet the diagnostic criteria for gender dysphoria – a strong rejection of typically feminine toys and clothes, mostly male friends; a sense that my feelings and reactions were typical of boys and the desire to be treated as a boy."

Following her detransition, in 2019 she set up the Detransition Advocacy Network, which in fewer than three months received more than 300 messages from young women regretting their transition.

---

256. https://www.genethique.org/detransition-de-genre-un-phenomene-dampleur/

These testimonies, the list could go on and on, are heart-breaking for us doctors and psychologists, whose constant preoccupation throughout our practising lives has been to try, with limited resources and varying degrees of success, to help and support our patients, as did countless country and family doctors of yesteryear who would run to the call of their patients, to give them the best possible care based on expertise drawn from the science of the day (Mercier decision of 1936). Far be it from us to influence their lifestyles, whatever their choice. What has happened to some among us?

**Associations supporting detransitioners**

Charlie Evans, the former trans journalist, has set up the Detransition Advocacy Network[257] with the aim of unifying and raising the voice and profile of these people, so that they feel less alone.

> "Detransitioning is not a result of societal pressure, it's a personal decision that we make because we were looking for a solution where we wouldn't find one".

In recent years, other groups have sprung up to support and defend the rights of people experiencing detransitioning: DetransCanada[258], Detrans Voices[259], SexChangeRegret.com[260], and in Belgium, Post Trans[261],

---

257. https://pro-lgbt.ru/fr/6649/
258. https://i.redd.it/7pgcf77up8161.png
259. https://twitter.com/detrans_voices
260. Take back your life others have. You can, too. https://sexchangeregret.com/
261. https://post-trans.com/Temoignage-detransition-francais-6

Our Duty[262]. In 2018, Häggström, father of a victim of trans ideology, launched the initiative Gender Identity Challenge Sweden[263] (GENID) after observing a worrying trend.

> "Almost no mother or father dares to refuse their child consent for surgery. This wish is now rarely questioned, as many parents report that their children have broken off contact with them because other young trans people have advised them to do so on the Internet.
>
> Two parents had also reported that the Youth Protection Office had called them back because they had refused to address their child using the "correct pronoun". The network has around a hundred members who want to prevent doctors from continuing to carry out experiments on their children.
>
> Operations and hormone treatments are an experiment, there are no long-term scientific studies on the consequences of such interventions. Young people cannot therefore give their informed consent."[264]

GENID is calling for a minimum age of 25 for surgery. The association points out the obvious: **all these treatments are de facto experimental**, as they have not been the subject of randomised trials in this indication, nor of major observational studies to demonstrate the benefit of

262. https://ourduty.group/
263. Gender Identity Challenge https://genderchallenge.no/home-1/
264. The TransTrain, Swedish Documentary with English subtitles https://www.youtube.com/watch?v=3lMa8ph_Xrs

these major treatments versus abstention and follow-up. These groups testify to the need of detransitioner communities to have their specific requirements met and to be brought out of the isolation that they once again face.

### Detransitioning, a growing phenomenon that is hard to quantify

While the mainstream media talk a great deal about gender and transitioning, detransitioning is a subject that rarely receives media coverage. Its study is made difficult by the militancy of certain doctors and by a medical and psychological follow-up that is too brief (many detransitions are carried out late, sometimes ten years after the sex change) and woefully inadequate for the transsexuals treated. The problem is concealed by the active censorship on the part of transgender extremists of any study or meeting to do with detransitioning.

### A fascination for transgender ideology among some doctors[265]

According to psychologist Professor Céline Masson, these doctors are "*tempted to administer what they see as a miracle cure that provides short-term relief; an attractive solution given the difficulty of treating disorders such as anorexia, autism or 'latent psychoses*".

Child psychiatrist Dr Anne Perret condemns the "*fascination with these discourses around transidentity*" on the part of health professionals, with "*the rigours of clinical practice giving way to militancy*". The result is "*overly hasty*

265. https://www.genethique.org/detransition-de-genre-un-phenomene-dampleur/

*medical interventionism*" and a psychological barrier to objectively studying the long-term results.

**Follow-up for transgender people is too brief and inadequate**

As surgeons and oncologists and/or paediatric oncologists, we have cared for the patients we have treated (surgically or with chemotherapy followed by monitoring in the crucial years of follow-up) all our lives (including in retirement if they wish, as advisors and/or friends made over the decades). Apart from the enormous satisfaction of staying in touch with these people, whose lives we shared at such important moments, this was the only way of knowing whether our indications were good and the operations relevant to their medical and general future, their lives, their jobs, their families and their children.

This is what makes our profession so enriching, despite the difficulties we face in dealing with the severity of the diseases, the lived experiences of our patients, and the inevitable and painful failures. The same is true of all the oncologists, surgeons, radiotherapists, ENT and other specialists, and of all the reputable doctors we have met: they monitor the patients they treat and they evaluate their results to improve the care of new patients. It is simply part of their duty of care.

Curiously, it seems that too few doctors prescribing transitional hormone therapy and too few sex reassignment surgeons carry out careful, regular and prolonged follow-up of their patients! This is astonishing, and most likely reflects the nature of the carers who engage in this demanding and difficult specialty, wherein psychiatry

plays a major role that is all too often disregarded by carer and patient alike. Is there any research in this area? Are we talking unregulated clinical trials?
To date, no large-scale, long-term study has assessed the incidence of detransitioning and the rate of regret in patients who have received gender affirmation treatment, particularly minors, whether or not they have opted for detransitioning. And yet studies of transitions and detransitions are essential if scientific knowledge and the management of gender dysphoria are to be improved[266].

In Great Britain, a report by Hilary Cass[267][268] found that Tavistock's paediatric gender reassignment service had not carried out "*systematic and consistent collection of data*" and that its "*approach has not been subjected to some of the usual control measures that are typically applied when new or innovative treatments are introduced*".
In addition, doctors had felt "*under pressure to adopt an unquestioning affirmative approach*"[269]. This was "*at odds with the standard process of clinical assessment and diagnosis that they have been trained to undertake in all other clinical encounters*". The report led to the closure of the specialist service[270].

266. https://www.reuters.com/investigates/section/youth-in-transition/
267. « Pression sur les médecins, manque de contrôle… : Un rapport du NHS met en cause le Tavistock Centre ». https://www.genethique.org/pression-sur-les-medecins-manque-de-controle-un-rapport-du-nhs-met-en-cause-le-tavistock-centre/
268. https://cass.independent-review.uk/
269. Which promotes the "affirmation" of gender solely on the basis of an individual's feelings.
270. "The Tavistock Clinic's closure follows a damning report on ideological malpractice", The Times, 29.7.2022. https://segm.org/Tavistock-closure-the-times

And therein lies the rub. This "speciality" is different from all the others: unlike in all other disorders (requiring transplants, amputations, chemotherapy, etc.), the underage patient has the right to decide; his or her immediate opinion is decisive, without multidisciplinary discussion or psychological care. Psychological follow-up is highly optional, and follow-up of patients undergoing hormone therapy or surgery is highly variable. To the best of our knowledge, it seems that the requirement of a multidisciplinary team meeting (MDTM) has not reached this group of patients.

In Sweden, the first country in the world to permit sex reassignment treatments, a report by the National Health Authority revealed that one in three girls aged between 13 and 17 treated for gender dysphoria actually suffered from an anxiety disorder, another third from depression, one in five from attention deficit disorder with or without hyperactivity and one in seven from autism. Devastating.
The health agency decided in February 2022[271] *"to halt hormone therapy for minors, except in very rare cases"* and that *"mastectomies for teenage girls wanting to transition should be limited to a research setting"*. In December 2022, in a press release, the head of the Council, Thomas Linden, stated: *"The uncertain state of knowledge calls for caution."*

271. https://www.france24.com/en/live-news/20230208-sweden-puts-brakes-on-treatments-for-trans-minors

In the USA, studies have shown that no "gender clinic" systematically monitors the outcomes of the people it treats, nor does it collect exhaustive data on the medium- and long-term outcomes of transgender people.

## Censorship of studies on detransitioning is often violent

Pro-transgender extremists systematically oppose scientific investigations and debates on detransitioning, resorting to defamation and sometimes even violence.
At the 2017 Philadelphia Trans Health Conference[272], two planned round tables on detransitioning were cancelled by the organising committee for fear that things might "*get out of control*".
The same year, when British psychotherapist James Caspian wanted to write his thesis at Bath Spa University on "detransition", his proposal was rejected by the ethics committee because of the risk that "*attacks on social media may not be confined to the researcher but may involve the university*"[273]. This censorship was accepted by the authorities, who told him that his subject could be deemed "*politically incorrect*". Caspian took his case to the Royal Court in 2019, but the judge refused to consider his application. His lawyers are now taking the case to the EU Court of Human Rights and argue that Caspian had "*his right to access the court violated, his freedom to pursue legitimate academic research breached, and that the basis of the decision to interfere with his academic freedom discriminated against him*".

272. https://www.arcusfoundation.org/events/2017-philadelphia-trans-health-conference/
273. https://www.thepinknews.com/2021/02/09/james-caspian-transgender-trans-bath-spa-european-court-human-rights/

What better way not to know than to bury your head in the sand?

Instead of objectively addressing the issue of detransitioning and putting forward their arguments, trans extremists accuse those who do of "*disinformation*" and of being "*close to the extreme right*", and campaign to prevent any reporting on the subject[274], such as the Radio Télévision Suisse documentary by Mauro Losa and Sofia Pekmez. The documentary (*Détransition, ils ont changé de sexe et ils regrettent*)[275] was accused of being simplistic and biased[276], as was the current affairs programme *Nous, les Européens Enfants transgenres : l'heure du doute*, in a report by Frédérique Maillard-Laudisa and Giona Messina on 25 November 2022[277].
Transgender extremists have no hesitation in proclaiming publicly in *Libération*[278] or in Médiapart[279], and numer-

274. "No to weaponising the subject of detransitioning in public debate". https://renverse.co/infos-locales/article/non-a-l-instrumentalisation-de-la-question-de-la-detransition-dans-le-debat-3904
275. https://www.rts.ch/play/tv/temps-present/video/detransition-ils-ont-change-de-sexe-et-ils-regrettent?urn=urn:rts:video:13829282
276. https://www.heidi.news/sante/enfants-trans-la-rts-s-emploie-a-faire-peur-avec-un-reportage-reducteur-et-oriente
277. https://www.francetvinfo.fr/replay-magazine/france-2/nous-les-europeens/nous-les-europeens-du-vendredi-25-novembre-2022_5457211.html
278. https://www.liberation.fr/debats/2020/02/26/le-debat-sur-la-place-des-femmes-trans-n-a-pas-lieu-d-etre_1779708/
279. https://blogs.mediapart.fr/arya-meroni/blog/240220/au-dela-du-debat-sur-la-place-des-femmes-trans-dans-le-mouvement-feministe

ous other "leftwing" media outlets[280][281][282][283] that: "*The debate on the place of trans women is uncalled-for*", thereby demonstrating their contempt for debating ideas, without which there can be no democracy, and ultimately for transgender people and/or feminists, whose future is of little importance to them, and whom they use as political propaganda material.

**How can we prevent children who feel transgender from being mutilated?**

The problem is not that a certain number of people feel that they are of a different sex from that of their visible body; this has always been the case among a very small minority. For adults who are aware of the consequences, gender reassignment is their business and their personal choice must be respected.

However, it is utterly paradoxical that children who are not mature enough to drive a car, sign cheques or consent to sexual relations should consent to treatments that will destroy their fertility and irreversibly alter their body. The problem becomes acute when those in political power assert that this is "*the new normal*", and attempt to indoctrinate our children in schools and to marginalise, indeed punish and dismiss, all those who oppose this new religion or who simply wish to raise questions.

To raise a child, you have to listen to them, talk to them,

280. https://agauche.org/2020/03/01/tribune-le-debat-sur-la-place-des-femmes-trans-na-pas-lieu-detre/

281. https://toutesdesfemmes.fr/tribune/

282. https://lanticapitaliste.org/actualite/feminisme/tribune-le-debat-sur-la-place-des-femmes-trans-na-pas-lieu-detre

283. https://www.europe-solidaire.org/spip.php?article52211

be the model for whatever you are advocating, and offer them other models that raise their moral standards and turn them away from narcissistic self-centredness.

To protect our children, we must demand an objective assessment of the transgender practices that have been in place for decades and should therefore come with a track record of their outcomes, and affirm, as Sweden, Finland, Hungary, the UK and more than 20 US states have done, that this is an experiment reserved for duly informed adults.

# 9.
# Transgender people: prison, changing rooms and toilets

## Some societal consequences in everyday life

While the vast majority of people do not want to discriminate against transgender people, they do want to ensure the safety of women in private places (prisons, toilets, changing rooms in particular). The dilemma of having to choose between transgender rights and the safety of women is the burning issue of the day. Feminists find themselves plunged into new dilemmas that they had not anticipated.

## French law advocates for inclusivity[284] of transgender people in prison

Life for transgender people in prison is not easy, as French general inspector of prisons Dominique Simonnot re-

284. In effect, allowing trans women born male to be incarcerated in women's prisons and trans men born female to be incarcerated in men's facilities.

minds us, in a notice published in the *Journal officiel* of July 2021:

> "Currently, transgender people deprived of their liberty suffer numerous infringements of their fundamental rights, the accumulation of which is likely to constitute cruel, inhuman or degrading treatment as defined by the European Convention on Human Rights."

> "The process of searching a person to see what they look like anatomically must be banned. It is too harsh, horribly intrusive and terribly humiliating."

> "The quarters prisoners are assigned, how they are searched, or their ability to continue with their medical treatment are often problematic in places where the freedom of expression of their gender is often annihilated or limited [...] the lack of consistent follow-up by doctors, as well as the difficulties for prisoners to continue their hormone treatment."

She also believes that *"a transgender man with a vagina can be incarcerated with men, the only thing that counts is the person's self-determination"*.

But between theory and practice lies the denial of reality and its difficulties, even with all the goodwill in the world.
The understandable decision to improve prison conditions for the tiny transgender minority (0.1 % of the general population) must not lead to women in prison

being put at risk, as shown by the examples of foreign countries that have practised a policy of inclusion for transgender prisoners before us.

**Safety concerns for biological women in contact with transsexual women (born male)**

In England, Karen White[285], a 52-year-old transgender woman, who had not undergone sex reassignment surgery, raped four of her fellow inmates at New Hall women's prison in Wakefield, West Yorkshire[286].

And this is not the only case in England: in 2020, *The Times* reported six instances of sexual assaults on women by fellow prisoners who were born male, but who claimed to be trans women[287].

In the USA, the *New York Post* reported[288] in April 2022 on a rape that took place in Rikers prison in New York State.

> "Ramel Blount, a transgender Rikers inmate, raped a female inmate while in the women's section of the jail and has been sentenced to seven years"[289].

285. "Transgender inmate admits Wakefield jail sex offences". https://www.bbc.com/news/uk-england-leeds-45436953
286. « Emprisonnée dans une prison pour femmes, la transgenre viole ses codétenues ». https://www.francesoir.fr/societe-faits-divers/emprisonnee-dans-une-prison-pour-femmes-la-transgenre-viole-ses-codetenues
287. https://www.thetimes.co.uk/article/seven-sex-attacks-in-womens-jails-by-transgender-convicts-cx9m8zqpg
288. https://nypost.com/2022/04/26/how-bowing-to-the-trans-lobby-led-to-a-rikers-prison-rape/
289. https://nypost.com/2022/04/25/transgender-rikers-inmate-gets-7-years-for-raping-female-prisoner/

In Canada[290], the newspaper *La Presse*[291] reported the case of Steve Mehlenbacher, who began identifying as a woman in 2018, calling herself Samantha, and was thus able to be transferred in 2019 to Grand Valley, one of Canada's five women's prisons.
This hardened criminal created "*a trail of victims, many of whom were terrorised*" by her behaviour and "*repeated breaches of conditions*" throughout her prison career. "*Fellow inmates were quick to accuse her of lying about her gender identity in order to have sex with women.*"

Ivan Zinger, from the Office of the Correctional Investigator of Canada (federal prison ombudsman), [292] pointed out in his 2018-2019 report that the integration of transgender prisoners in women's prisons has been the subject of several complaints from female inmates[293].

> "The concern raised is understandable, particularly in light of the fact that most sentenced women have experienced significant trauma and sexual and physical violence in their lives."

> "In addition, we cannot completely ignore the fact that manipulation may be the reason why a male inmate might express a desire to live as a transgender."

290. https://www.courrierinternational.com/article/prisons-au-canada-des-derapages-lies-a-la-protection-des-detenues-transgenres
291. https://www.lapresse.ca/actualites/2022-10-01/transgenres-emprisonnees-avec-des-femmes/cohabitation-controversee.php#
292. Swedish term meaning people's representative.
293. https://www.lapresse.ca/actualites/2022-10-01/transgenres-emprisonnees-avec-des-femmes/cohabitation-controversee.php

Members of the Union of Federal Correctional Officers fear transgender transfers because they feel they are not equipped to deal with them.

In Scotland, Isla Bryson born Adam Graham, convicted of raping two women in 2016 and 2019, began her gender transition between her crimes and her trial. Her temporary incarceration in a women's institution sparked public outrage,[294] eventually leading to a change in policy. Transgender prisoners are now incarcerated in a prison appropriate to their birth gender.

In Denmark, the Eastern High Court ruled on appeal that a transgender woman (born male) who changed her gender while in prison for aggravated rape, but who did not undergo surgical transition, must serve her sentence in a male institution[295], because her presence in a women's prison *"would pose a significant security risk to women prisoners"*.

The High Court ruled that the fact that the prisoner was *"strip-searched by men"* and had to *"provide a urine sample"* under the supervision of men did not breach the Execution of Sentences Act, as the reference to gender in the Act must be *"understood as biological sex"*.

As rape of all kinds is a notorious prison problem, there is nothing transphobic about refusing to house people with

294. "Isla Bryson: Transgender rapist jailed for eight years". https://www.bbc.com/news/uk-scotland-64796926

295. https://www.leparisien.fr/societe/danemark-une-femme-transgenre-non-operee-doit-rester-dans-sa-prison-pour-hommes-24-05-2023-G3MCJZH4XRGPVICKLTQKS2Y2JU.php

male genitalia in a women's unit. Refusing to acknowledge concrete biological facts in such cases simply puts female prisoners at risk.

**Transgender people in dormitories**

The headache faced by boarding school headmasters is similar to that faced by prison governors. In France, the Education Minister's circular on boarding schools states that the school *"may authorise the pupil to occupy a room in a part of the school that conforms to his or her identity"*, but does not specify what to do when no solution that respects both women by birth and trans women is possible. It is up to the headmaster to deal with the consequences whichever way it goes!

The problem was starkly illustrated by the mother of a trans boy (born a girl) who had not undergone an operation and was staying in the girls' dormitory during a week's holiday camp. "*He came back very traumatised. He couldn't bear to go to school for a week, and we had to help him digest the humiliation and the rejection he'd experienced*", said the mother, who accused Puteaux Municipality of transphobia[296]. The Municipality replied that they "*obviously wanted what was best for this child, but also for others*". They explained that a single room was requested for Léo from the service provider, but that none was available.

Does the mother realise that placing her child with female

296. https://rmc.bfmtv.com/actualites/societe/education/son-fils-dans-le-dortoir-des-filles-pendant-une-colo-elle-accuse-la-ville-de-puteaux-de-transphobie_AV-202303130475.html

genitalia in a boys' dormitory in these violent times would have exposed him to mockery, inappropriate gestures and even gang rape? There is again a denial of reality despite the good intentions. Conversely, placing a young trans girl (born male) who has not undergone surgery in a girls' dormitory would constitute a threat to the girls.

The solution found at Caen prison to create a section reserved for transgender people - is it the best one, as well as for all boarding schools?
The safety of a trans minor clearly cannot be guaranteed in a dormitory of the opposite sex, and it is not transphobic to prioritise their safety over their inclusion.
What's more, the ministerial circular advocating the inclusion of transgender pupils on school trips and outings specifies that this should be applied "*as far as possible*". Get on with it and don't rock the boat. Thank you, Minister.
Let's hope that on this issue, wisdom will prevail over ideology, and that judges will be able to use the formula of the Danish Court of Appeal as to prisons: "*The reference to gender in the law must be understood as biological sex.*"

**Transgender people and changing rooms**

For a transgender person, the gym and changing rooms can be terrifying. Thus, the law requires that they should have access to facilities according to their gender.
Let's not forget that the vast majority of them are fragile people whose depression, autistic tendencies or other psychological disorders have not been taken into account, everything being put down to "gender dysphoria". But their behavioural problems and suffering are there for

all to see, and their extreme sensitivity is omnipresent. Since nothing has in fact been solved, any exposure to a risk linked to their gender - on which they have banked everything, because they believed in the promised miracle cure - is cruel, hence the recurrent issue of the "changing rooms" at school, in sporting facilities, etc. We must not underestimate the reality of their experiences in this respect, the terrible situations in which they have been trapped without considering their underlying psychological state: a real problem, in fact, that should be taken seriously and not seen as play-acting.

When schools, as they are authorised to do so, "*agree with the pupil on the introduction of flexible timetables*" for his/her use of changing facilities, the application of the law does not seem to pose any major problems in terms of security and privacy.
But in the real world, disturbing examples abound of men taking advantage of inclusive policies to enter girls' changing rooms as they wish. Between the suffering of trans individuals who must be respected and the criminal manipulation of the situation by unscrupulous individuals, we must not be naïve.
The Young Men's Christian Association (YMCA) defends an extremely inclusive policy instituted by the State of California, whereby any trans person who is not recognised as a sexual aggressor can use the changing rooms of the gender to which they claim to belong without restriction. In January 2023, during a trip to San Diego organised by the YMCA, Rebecca Phillips, a minor who was showering in the girls' changing rooms, was confronted by a naked man

claiming to be a trans woman[297]. In protest, parents have come together to form "SanteeParents4Choice" and have organised a rally for women's and girls' rights to ensure that such an incident cannot happen again.

**How the pronouncements of some sectarian ideologues are harmful to sportsmen and women**

Abbigail Wheeler, 16, a swimmer with the Springfield YMCA SPY swim team, was banned from the YMCA and expelled from her swim team for objecting to a naked man in their women's changing room,[298] after being accused of "hate speech". Her older sister had previously experienced exactly the same thing with Lia Thomas.

In New York, Ali Miles, a transgender woman (born male), decided to sue a yoga studio that forced her to use the men's changing rooms, after her presence caused an uproar and led to complaints from other customers in the women's changing rooms[299]. A witness to the scene told the *New York Post*:

> "This person who claims to be a transitioning woman came into the female locker room, in male shorts that were down to his knees. [...] he did not wear any feminine top to cover his bust [...] He was crouched down on the

297. https://nypost.com/2023/01/14/sighting-of-trans-womans-penis-in-ymca-locker-room-sparks-tears/
298. https://www.washingtontimes.com/news/2023/jul/13/support-grows-abbigail-wheeler-who-was-booted-swim/
299. https://www.demotivateur.fr/article/une-femme-transgenre-poursuit-un-studio-de-yoga-apres-avoir-ete-forcee-d-utiliser-les-vestiaires-des-hommes-34223

> floor in front of the shower stalls. It was very uncomfortable for one of the women that was in there and she as completely naked."

Ali Miles is claiming $5 million in damages.

To alleviate the discomfort that all students - transgender and cisgender - might feel in such contexts, new changing rooms should be designed with privacy in mind, with individual showers, changing cubicles and toilets that are private and enclosed. This would promote the well-being not only of transgender athletes, but also of any athlete with a preference for modesty.

**Transgender people and toilets**

Access to toilets is one of the concerns most often raised by transgender people[300]. They describe feelings of discomfort, stress and anxiety combined with anger about using public toilets[301].

They are aware that holding back urine is bad for their health, but using public toilets seems riskier for them. Transgender men (born female) often feel they need a companion to accompany them to the toilet to reduce

300. Hardacker C. T., Baccellieri A., Mueller E. R., Brubaker L., Hutchins G., Zhang J. L. Y., Hebert-Beirne J. "Bladder Health Experiences, Perceptions and Knowledge of Sexual and Gender Minorities". Int J Environ Res Public Health. 2019 Aug. 30; 16(17):3170. doi: 10.3390/ijerph16173170. PMID: 31480302; PMCID: PMC6747507. https://www.ncbi.nlm.nih.gov/pmc/articles/PMC6747507/

301. Rood B. A., Reisner S. L., Surace F. I., Puckett J. A., Maroney M. R., Pantalone D. W. "Expecting Rejection: Understanding the Minority Stress Experiences of Transgender and Gender-Nonconforming Individuals". *Transgend Health.* 2016 Aug. 1; 1(1):151-164. doi: 10.1089/trgh.2016.0012. PMID: 29159306; PMCID: PMC5685272.

the risk of violence, and they prefer to travel to places where they can access safe toilets.
Avoidance of toilets out of rejection of dirt or fear for their safety leads to urinary problems such as "weaker bladders".

An experiment with unisex toilets in a secondary school in Seine-Saint-Denis and another in Bordeaux became the cause for self-congratulation by the school management and pro-trans organisations alike.

> "By renovating the toilets, making them mixed sex and putting in place new rules for use, we are taking action for cleaner toilets, so that pupils don't have to hold back anymore and for a calmer atmosphere within the school".

But the overwhelmingly negative reactions expressed online contradict this opinion.

It is difficult to understand how making toilets unisex can make the atmosphere in a school more serene. It may reduce the waiting time for females, who regularly have to queue for their loos, but increase it for boys and men who are deprived of urinals to the delight of certain trans activists who see them as *"flashy instruments of toxic masculinity"*.
In fact, the principal of a school in Bordeaux admits that[302]: *"I'm all for fighting against determinism, and I'm all for equality between men and women, but in this case, I don't see what good it does."*

302. https://www.sudouest.fr/gironde/marsas/gironde-les-toilettes-non-genrees-pas-encore-dans-les-moeurs-a-marsas-6172388.php

Everyone wants safe, private, lockable and clean toilets. It's hard to understand why the management of these establishments waited so long to renovate, maintain and clean them properly. But making them mixed sex only pleases a tiny insecure minority.

**Conclusions**

The appropriation of places that used to be reserved for women, such as dormitories, changing rooms, showers, toilets and shelters by biological men who call themselves trans women gives men ever more power and the ability to break down all the protections that women have fought for.

Let's salute the common sense of UK Prime Minister Rishi Sunak in his statement on 13 April 2023:

> "We should always have compassion and understanding and tolerance for those who are thinking about changing their gender, but when it comes to these issues of protecting women's rights and women's spaces, as a general operating principle for me, biological sex is vitally, fundamentally important - we can't forget that - and that's why we need to make sure, particularly when it comes to women's health, women's sports or indeed women's spaces, that we're protecting those rights and those places."

# 10.
# The gender business: a multi-billion-dollar market

**Financial profiteering under the guise of humanism and a clear conscience?**
According to a study by Market Watch, the US market for sex reassignment surgery was worth \$1.9 billion in 2021. With an annual growth rate of 11 %, it should reach \$6 billion in 2030. This is not to be sniffed at, even under the guise of good intentions.

For some surgeons bored with the routine of an appendicitis or fractured hip surgery, sexual transformation surgery can be a distraction, even an attraction, as it also gives them a measure of fame[303] and significant financial gains, and perhaps even, in the best of cases, an opportunity to show off their creativity. Some clin-

303. Such as having your name appear in the list of "the World's best transgender surgeons" https://www.clinicspots.com/fr/blog/best-transgender-doctors

ics have developed this activity into a highly lucrative model.

The Philadelphia Center for Transgender Surgery has published some of the prices charged by its surgeons: $25,600 for so-called bottom surgery[304], almost $60,000 for "top" surgery, i.e. thoracic surgery, and more than $70,000 for facial reconstruction. This puts the price of surgery alone at around $124,400 for female-to-male transition and $140,450 for male-to-female transition.

Vanderbilt University's paediatrics transgender clinic "raises serious moral, ethical and legal concerns", said Tennessee Republican Governor Bill Lee. Its surgical activities are highly lucrative: $40,000 for female-to-male "chest reconstruction", $20,000 for vaginoplasty, and up to $100,000 for complete female-to-male surgical transformations. Matt Walsh[305] posted a video online showing Dr Shayne Taylor talking about the lucrative aspects of transgender surgeries: "Some of our financial people at VUMC (Vanderbilt University Medical Centre) in October 2016 put down some costs of how much money we think each patient will bring in ... and that's a lot of money."

Walsh observed that management paid trans activists to educate staff and attend transgender patient appointments to monitor doctors and prevent "dangerous" behaviour such as misgendering.

The clinic's management muzzled opposition from its

---

304. Terms like "bottom" or "top surgery" are used around young people as this terminology is deemed less harsh and more acceptable and it is therefore used by surgeons too.

305. https://www.dailysignal.com/2022/09/21/vanderbilt-tennessee-governor-lee-matt-walsh-transgender-surgeries-minors/

doctors through "threats and coercion" and as Dr Ellen Clayton, speaking at a conference in November 2019, put it[306], it "should not be without consequence" if some of the doctors objected to transgender surgeries, such as vaginoplasties and phalloplasties, being carried out on patients[307]. These revelations have convinced Vanderbilt University, which is being investigated for potential medical billing fraud[308] to discontinue the clinic's transgender activities. As well as surgery at absurd prices, prescribing drugs for life is a source of income both for prescribers, who secure a captive clientele, and for pharmaceutical companies, who can also manipulate prices, since patients are dependent on these drugs. Are people warned of this before making any decisions ? Are teenagers capable of detecting all the traps hidden behind the apparent philanthropy of influencers and complicit doctors ?

Gender theory leads to "*the commodification of children's bodies*"[309] and turns them into "*lifelong consumers of hormonal chemicals marketed by pharmaceutical companies*". In the USA, the cost of drugs and surgery can reach $200,000 for a single "patient"[310].

306. https://www.faithwire.com/2022/09/21/vanderbilt-faces-intense-backlash-over-pediatric-transgender-clinic-doctor-says-those-who-object-should-face-consequences/
307. https://generationsnouvelles.net/le-centre-medical-de-luniversite-vanderbilt-suspend-les-operations-transgenres-pour-les-enfants-apres-un-rapport/
308. https://francedaily.news/fr/lhopital-vanderbilt-remet-les-dossiers-de-la-clinique-transgenre-au-procureur-general-du-gop-dans-le-cadre-dune-enquete/161596.html
309. https://www.lantieditorial.fr/episode/enfants-transgenres-est-on-alle-trop-loin/
310. https://www.insider.com/medical-treatments-transgender-people-america-expensive-2019-7

Faced with an "*increase in gender dysphoria*", American insurance companies such as Aetna and Unicare are agreeing to cover the costs of certain types of operation in adults : removal of the ovaries and fallopian tubes, hysterectomy or removal of the testicles.
The cost of puberty blockers, such as GnRH agonists, can be prohibitive for patients : the estimated cost of paediatric leuprolide (injection every three months) is around $9,500 and that of the drug histrelin is $39,000[311]. Understandably, pharmaceutical companies actively support transgender rights organisations.
So, in addition to the amount charged for surgery, the running costs for maintaining your chosen gender are often high, as Claire, an American trans woman, explains :

> "The most expensive thing for a trans woman is hair removal : about $75 to $150 per session just for your face. And you may need to do that for three to seven years.
> Before chest surgery, you also have to use binders (at $40 each) to keep your breasts from being so visible, and there are plenty of other expenses that most people never have to think about. I probably have spent upward over $200,000, maybe $300,000, in just medical."

The pharmaceutical and medical industries must have better patient engagement to achieve better outcomes. This was the conclusion of a report published by PwC Health Research Institute (HRI) called "Patient Engage-

311. Salas-Humara C., Sequeira G. M., Rossi W., Dhar C. P. "Gender affirming medical care of transgender youth". *Curr Probl Pediatr Adolesc Health Care.* 2019 Sep. ; 49(9):100683 Epub, 2019 Nov. 15.

ment: Pharma's Strategy for Success in the New Health Economy".

Patient engagement is vital for the pharmaceutical industry, as customers are taking charge of their wellbeing independent of pharmaceuticals and are demanding to be more involved in their own healthcare decisions. This has resulted in highly targeted and seductive advertising and an inexhaustible "beauty" market. Gender theory is not just a humanistic, progressive gimmick, but a monstrous commodification of the body under the false banner of compassion, care and psychology. One hell of a business.

# 11.
# Social networks

How much responsibility do social networks have in the reported "epidemic" of gender dysphoria (or, more accurately, in the significant increase in the number of people who identify as transgender) ?

Very often blamed for all the problems of our time, and in particular for the decline in the general level of education, social networks, like computers and all digital devices, are merely tools. In fact, as in so many areas, these tools are responsible for both the best and the worst. The best is, after all, a certain resistance to the woke hegemony of the mainstream audiovisual and print media. These are owned by fewer than a dozen billionaires and enable them to launch slogans that will be repeated worldwide using the same words and images in every language at the same time. This stratagem convinces people that "everyone agrees" and thus paves the way for submission.

Is the "epidemic" of sex reassignment requests purely the result of shameless online propaganda, exacerbated by the greed of unethical professionals and highly profitable private establishments? Can social networks, which are often accused of all kinds of things, really take some, if not all, of the blame for this?

The answer is yes, in part. We have seen that gender theory has its most important roots in the 1960s of last century, well before the Internet really became a popular tool (which we can date from around 2000-2010). Social networks did not create the phenomenon but allowed it to be amplified.

At a time when globalist powers are trying to impose an all-digital approach to administrative services, schools, universities and healthcare, the role of social networks has become very significant. The great global experiment of the "lockdowns" revealed their limits, but also their usefulness in countering the monopoly on truth. The moral of the story is that the networks give us a certain freedom that has allowed the best and the worst to flourish (and they make the leaders of Western governments and the EU throw fits of rage from sheer powerlessness).

**The real role of networks (TikTok, Instagram, etc.)**

Testimonies abound of the strong pressure put on teenagers by LGBTQ+ lobbies via social networks (preferably those least frequented by adults), to encourage them to "assert themselves" and impose their difference.

For many young people who are feeling unhappy, these sudden signs of attention from groups who say they understand them seem kind and consoling (unlike their parents, who might refuse any discussion and who are, in their view, from another time).

The pro-gender groups instantly accept them, comfort them, charm them, seduce them and in effect hold them under their sway, very much like classic narcissistic perverts. Seduction is followed by brutal rejection if the person wants to break away. So, they stay, preferring kindness and the appearance of love to insults and disparagement, especially as they have become a public figure, easy to harass on a variety of media if they try to escape this hold[312].

Parents are generally left out of the process and are unaware of it for a long time. When they finally find out, they don't know how to react, or how to avoid the sometimes-serious consequences of hasty decisions (family break-up, the teenager fleeing to his room or away from home, sometimes risking homelessness). What's more, they could find themselves under the critical eye of the social services, who are quickly informed of the situation (by whom ?) if they don't respond enthusiastically to their offspring's sudden wishes.

Here are a few thoughts on the role of social networks, inspired by the testimonies of young people in turmoil[313]. Over the last three years or so, the phenomenon known as gender dysphoria has worsened dramatically as a re-

312. All the books on bullying in the family or in the workplace by narcissistic perverts can help to understand how this general pattern is reproduced. See, for example, the work of psychiatrist Geneviève Pagnard, a specialist in the subject.

313. https://odysee.com/@Impellobel.odysee:b/Dysphorie-de-GENRE--le-mirage-de-la-TRANSITION:6?

sult of the disastrous lockdowns of 2020 which have left teenagers glued to their laptops or computers, deprived of normal social and amicable relationships in the real world (particularly at the time of adolescence and the first stirrings of love) and this has given free rein to all possible excesses, with no limits. A profusion of videos in a wide variety of fields have replaced the reading of actual books with commentary by teachers. They have led to cognitive dissonance in young people in particular, who are on the receiving end of a deluge of fanciful notions in science, medicine, psychology or parapsychology, etc., amid real scientific information. Immersed in all this jumble (parents-now has-beens, teachers now marginalised, sidelined, overwhelmed), how could anyone cope?
The stage was set for predators of every ilk, including sex and all its variations. Are you unhappy? Then you're in the wrong body. We'll sort it out…
Influencers in search of customers, emerging at this time to fill a professional and/or friendship void, assumed a very special importance in the lives of these young people who were deprived of school, and sometimes at loggerheads with their parents because of forced lockdowns and permanent over-crowding at home that would soon become unbearable. Breaking up families, one of the aims of the globalists, had now acquired an additional tool and undeniable success…
As for the malaise (=dysphoria) linked to gender, it has worsened in France since these troubled times.
Some teachers report having been confronted with the type of pattern already described in the USA, whereby, all of a sudden, in the space of a few days, a group of

young girls calling themselves boys is formed. They know each other, are close friends or classmates. There's a social contagion that gives them a feeling of belonging to a group.

At last, no longer being alone, or at least no longer feeling alone thanks to the group that you can find whenever you want online, without censorship, without limits, 24 hours a day. Exchanges can last for hours on the laptop hidden under the covers.

These young girls sometimes spur each other on by fear of their own femininity. The challenges of being a woman today mean that many young girls no longer dress as they choose, but as a preventive measure to limit attacks in the metro, and they no longer visit certain areas or streets in large cities such as Paris.

Pornography, which is so widespread on the Internet and easily viewed by preadolescents at a very young age, leads to a mental intrusion that upsets them, and also to a certain rejection of femininity by young girls who are disgusted by what they have seen.

Very often, these young girls are from well-off families and their mothers, who are liberal and frequently absent, have passed on a victim-based feminism to their daughters. "*As women, they will always be victims*". What's more, they have an image of sexuality as being brutal, not only through the image of women in pornographic films, but also through stories of feminicide and of a society that no longer punishes rape, even when it is repeated. So, isn't it better to be a man? But is that what we call feeling like a man?

The lectures at school explain, against all historical evidence, that "*as women, they have always been victims since time began*". So, since the myth of gender theory tells them that the notion of woman is purely and simply a construct, that there is a patriarchal plot to impose heterosexuality, why not choose the right gender?

When the ground is well prepared and fertilised, the influencers[314] refer them to militant doctors and/or provide them with addresses where they can buy hormone modifiers without medical supervision.
The advantage of social networks is that they can pass on positive recruitment messages, just as they do in sects. People who make the transition experience a moment of euphoria. Among them are real patients with pathologies who should have been treated by real psychiatrists: "*people who can only shower in the dark. They feel liberated*". But for how long? When the unhappiness inevitably returns (because the underlying problem has not been tackled), the young victims are once again alone and lost.

## Confusion between homosexuality and transgenderism

On social networks, we can see many young girls who want to become boys initially identify themselves as lesbians. But these are very different things.
Many testimonies show that they are quickly pushed to "change their gender" and that there is no protection online for the militant effect: "no safeguards": "*I am what I say I am*", "*It's a given that cannot be discussed*", they are

314. Not necessarily financially disinterested!

told. The people who come back from this experience have the impression that they are escaping from the grip of a sect-like group. Adolescents in thrall to the Internet have effectively excluded themselves from their families, isolating themselves from them and refusing to communicate. They replace these all-important ties with the influence of gurus who tell them what to do and, above all, what to think.

The digitisation of communications intensified and promoted by the Covid "plandemic", has multiplied these dramatic dangers for our young people. Glued to their mobile phones at all times, they forget that man is a social animal who, without human contact, particularly physical contact, degenerates[315]. Influencers flood them with overly affectionate and often sham messages. But woe betide those who hesitate, the renegades who feel they've made a mistake. They are insulted, defamed and even harassed by the very same people. If they take a step backwards, they become traitors to the cause, reactionary, worthless. Imagine the psychological devastation for these already fragile teenagers.

Parents must regain their protective authority against all this propaganda from the media, films, schools and universities, to give their children guidelines and limits. A child, and then a teenager, needs to feel this benevolent force close to him, not the power of oppression that can-

315. The "Free Hugs" sessions organised on the Promenade des Anglais after the unjust coercive measures came to an end reinvigorated many of them. Embracing passers-by was enough to restore contact, a breath of fresh air and a desire to live. Simply touching them is a human gesture that everyone needs, just like holding the hand of an elderly person lying in bed. Well done to the woman who inaugurated these moments of healing in Nice.

cel culture would have us believe, but the power of love. By doing away with the image of the father and seeking to replace it with state medical paternalism, on the pretext of medical prevention, the globalists have dismantled parental authority.

# 12.
# Propaganda, censorship and backlash

**Transgenderism as a source of power**

Feminism has become outdated and no longer pays off in terms of advancement to the highest echelons of society, because the good jobs are already taken. Something else had to be found. For several years now, the media, official bodies and the Internet have been engaging in intense pro-gender and pro-transsexual propaganda aimed officially at promoting "inclusiveness", while in practice acceding to their wish for greater visibility[316] by giving transgender people more jobs at all levels of the workforce.

This, it is worth noting, is the opinion of only a minority of transgender people as the majority, like everyone else, wants to live in peace and quiet without attracting attention. It seems though that the most vocal adherents are more concerned with obtaining prestigious positions

316. Some have been very successful, like Joe Biden's Deputy Secretary of Health, for example.

under this banner than with their gender, their transgenderism being merely a means of gaining access to power. This media propaganda, coupled with that of the same lobbies on social networks, has gone hand-in-hand with an increase in gender dysphoria (discomfort) among young people and is creating a boomerang effect of intolerance towards sexual minorities, with a net increase in homophobic and transphobic acts.
Isn't it time for a more measured and cautious approach to the over-representation of transgender people, in the interests of sexual minorities who have hitherto been fairly well accepted by the population?

**Pro-trans propaganda is omnipresent**
Gender dysphoria was included as a diagnosis in the latest edition of the American manual of mental disorders (DSM-5-TR)[317]. Over the course of the various editions of this manual, the expressions applied to it have changed from *transsexualism to gender incongruence and subsequently gender dysphoria.*
Since 2013, the American Psychiatric Association (APS) has stated that "*gender dysphoria is not a mental disorder*", and the WHO did the same in 2019. The APS estimates the incidence to be 0.005 % to 0.014 % of people born male and 0.002 % to 0.003 % of people born female. It is not a new condition, but since 2017 it has received a lot of media attention, as the following chart from the French language dictionary shows[318].

317.https://www.msdmanuals.com/fr/professional/troubles-psychiatriques/sexualité-dysphorie-de-genre-et-paraphilies/incongruence-et-dysphorie-de-genre
318. https://www.lalanguefrancaise.com/dictionnaire/definition/dysphorie-de-genre

Frequency in which the French word for "gender dysphoria" has appeared in World's newpapers

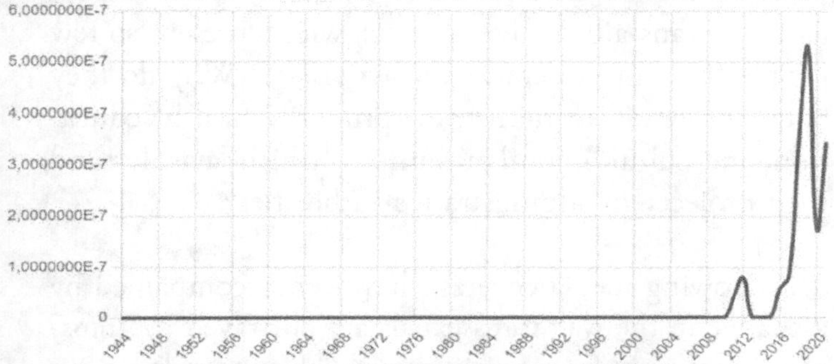


Source: Gallicagram. Developed by Benjamin Azoulay and Benoît de Courson, Gallicagram plots the trend over time in the use of a syntagm

At the same time, there has been an explosion in the number of medical articles, mainly American, published each year on the subject[319].

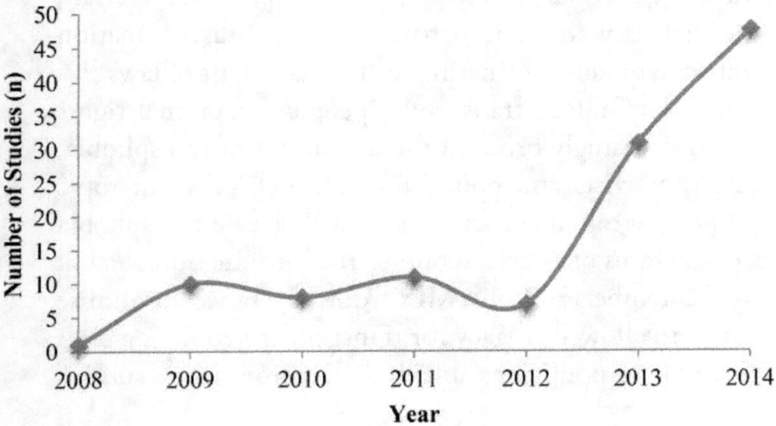


319. Reisner S. L., Poteat T., Keatley J., Cabral M., Mothopeng T., Dunham E., Holland C. E., Max R., Baral S. D. "Global health burden and needs of transgender populations: a review". *Lancet.* 2016 Jul. 23; 388(10042):412-436. *Epub* 2016 June 17. https://www.ncbi.nlm.nih.gov/pmc/articles/PMC7035595/

Why do the public authorities attach so much importance to trans-affirmative activists, who represent so few people (first and foremost the activists!)? Why do they open the doors to ministries (primarily health, education, and culture), local authorities, which lavishly fund their projects, or administrative authorities?

This growing media coverage has been accompanied by a change in the way transsexuals are portrayed[320]. Transgenderism went from being a marginal issue in the 1980s (transvestites and transsexuals, particularly Brazilians in the Bois de Boulogne park in Paris) to becoming a "social phenomenon" in the 1990s (the popularisation of transgender cabaret), then a "social issue" (illness or condition?), now a *major societal problem* exploited by certain politicians who see it as part of the anti-discrimination movement, all culminating in the enactment of laws[321]. These laws afford transgender people exceptional rights and increasingly broaden the definitions of transphobia. Trans activists and politicians in search of a hot topic hope to create a consensus that will elevate transphobia to the status of a social scourge. The introduction of a bill in September 2023 by MPs from La France Insoumise Party to allow surrogacy for transgender people is a clear example of politicians able to deflect from issues such as

320. « Les constructions médiatiques des personnes trans – Un exemple d'inscription dans le programme « Penser le genre » en SIC. » https://www.cairn.info/revue-les-enjeux-de-l-information-et-de-la-communication-2014-1-page-35.htm

321. On 18 November 2016, the "21st Century Justice Modernisation Act" was passed, according to which it is possible to change your gender on your identity papers, if you are perceived by those around you to be of the gender by which you define yourself.

soaring poverty or the loss of freedom of expression. The manipulation of these suffering transgender people by politicians is highly shocking and demonstrative of the patient as objectified citizen.

To claim, as some extremist trans activists do, that "*reducing gender to biological sex forms the basis of transphobic discourse*" shows the degree they have reached in their denial of reality and their bigotry. Let us remind them that transphobia is defined by an expressed rejection, contempt or hatred towards transgender people, and not by a reminder of the indisputable biological fact that humanity is bisexual, like all evolved living species.

## Extensive, unfounded but intimidating accusations of transphobia

In Canada, it was recently reported that a pupil accused of being transphobic was expelled from his school for saying that there were only two biological sexes[322]. Dave Bloch, a snowboarding coach at Woodstock Union High School where he had worked for ten years, was dismissed from his job for intervening in a conversation between two pupils about whether a man who claimed to be a woman could legitimately compete against women. He said that in his opinion men differed from women genetically, and that this gave them an advantage in sport, being statistically faster and stronger, and was sacked for expressing his opinion[323]. Dismissed by authorities in de-

---

322. https://www.msn.com/fr-fr/actualite/education/un-%C3%A9l%C3%A8ve-canadien-d-une-%C3%A9cole-catholique-exclu-de-son-lyc%C3%A9e-pour-avoir-dit-qu-il-n-y-avait-que-deux-genres/ar-AA17kG0g

323. https://www.washingtontimes.com/news/2023/jul/19/david-bloch-snowboarding-coach-sues-school-after-b/

nial. We showed in the chapter on transgender sport that he was merely reporting facts that are now recognised by most international sports federations.

Geneviève de Fontenay[324], patron of the Miss France pageant for decades, was indicted on charges of "transphobic insults" after pointing out that article 2 of the pageant regulations stipulates that "Candidates for the title of Miss France must not have undergone plastic surgery", thereby reserving candidacies for natural-born women only, no trans woman having yet entered such a pageant without having undergone multiple operations. What a terrible end to the career of a woman who had given her all to this legendary competition.

The fear on the part of families, psychiatrists, general and other medical practitioners of being prosecuted for transphobia if they refuse to immediately comply with a child's wish to come out and receive treatments designed to transform them means that too many minors jump on board the high-speed train to transition, without the benefit of a long period for their decision to mature along with their family, teachers and family doctors. Ultimately, these children are victims of the fashions imposed by the lobbies, and will pay the price for the rest of their lives.

This very small sexual minority (0.02 to 0.1 % of the population) is often featured in television series, films,

---

324. https://www.ohmymag.com/people/actu-people/genevieve-de-fontenay-mise-en-examen-pour-transphobie-ses-propos-choquants-tenus-en-2021_art159461.html

documentaries, websites, symposia, publications and artistic works, sometimes with no justification either artistically or in the storyline, to increase its visibility. Since December 2020, four documentaries and reports promoting gender theory and/or trans sexualism have been broadcast on the Arte, M6, TMC and TF1 channels in France, some of them in prime time, i.e. during family time in front of the TV.

### Promoting sex reassignment, a "left-wing" political identifier

Former Education Minister Pap Ndiaye has proclaimed that "*sex education in schools is my priority*" and claimed that "*teaching gender theory in schools would combat discrimination, sexual and sexist violence and LGBT phobia*". Under the guise of sex education, the Ministry has organised the promotion of gender theory and transsexualism in schools by grant-funded associations. In September 2021 (by Minister Jean-Michel Blanquer under pressure), it issued a circular for schools to affirm a child's self-determined gender. This transidentity propaganda in schools is convincing more and more children that they may have been born in the wrong body, that it is up to them to choose whether to be a girl or a boy, and that it is possible to change "gender" and sex! Unfortunately, feelings of unease among pre-teens and teenagers are a normal part of the transition to adulthood. The increasing reduction of such feelings to problems of identification means that depression and other psychological and psychiatric disorders (exacerbated by lockdowns and coercive measures during the Covid period) are being over-

looked and that a false diagnosis is being used as a sticking-plaster that leaves them isolated in their suffering.
Promoted by the media and showbiz, supported by the State and the international courts, the claims of transsexual rights are widely exploited by political activists and are the latest fashion in progressive struggles. After abandoning the poorest classes - blue-collar, white-collar and low-wage workers - parties in search of new constituencies have specialised in defending minorities, importing the American story into France, one that is not our own. The proliferation in universities of meetings purportedly held to combat racism but "off-limits to white people" speaks to the current madness in a country that for so long was not racist. The defence of sexual minorities, hitherto widely accepted, is part of a political and electoral calculation in which these same minorities sometimes become the collateral victims.
Joe Biden chose Rachel Levine, a trans woman, as his Assistant Health Secretary:

> "She is a historic and deeply qualified choice to help lead our administration's health efforts. ... she will bring the steady leadership and essential expertise we need to get people through this pandemic."

This primarily political choice was intended to confirm his "progressivism" in order to secure the votes of the radical leftists in his party. Democrats are more than four times as likely as Republicans to say that a person's gender can be different from the gender they were assigned at birth (61 % versus 13 %) and also much more likely than Republicans to say that our society has not gone far enough in accepting transgender people (59 % versus 10 %). Meanwhile, 66 % of Republicans say society has gone too far in accepting transgender people.

In France too, "*communication on identity is used to pander to certain electoral constituencies and especially the left of the party*", admits Lauric Henneton, lecturer at the University of Versailles Saint-Quentin, "*we can only imagine that it's an American version of the French satirical film 'En même temps*'."

In 2022, Andy Kerbrat, France Insoumise MP for Loire-Atlantique, together with a hundred or so elected politicians and left-wing activists, launched a petition "***For a government without LGBTQIA+ phobias***" demanding "the resignation" of Caroline Cayeux, Minister Delegate for Territorial Cohesion; Christophe Béchu, Minister of Ecology and Gérald Darmanin, Minister of the Interior, by calling them "notorious LGBTQIA+ phobes".
Most psychiatrists and surgeons talk of "*an insane response to an insane demand*", accusing the media of giving the subject too much publicity and, as a result, "*fostering career opportunities*".

**The "transsexual "epidemic**
The relatively large increase in the number of transsexuals who have followed this propaganda shows that it has been effective. Thirty years ago, there were 3,000 trans-

sexuals in Germany; today there are 24,000. In France[325], the overall prevalence of gender dysphoria has increased more than 9-fold in seven years (from 1.5/100,000 in 2013 to 14/100,000 in 2020), particularly in the under-17s (+3,575 %).

Similar increases in incidence have been observed in most Western countries: "Depending on the country, over a period of ten to fifteen years, diagnoses have risen by between 1,000 % and 4,000 %"[326]. It should be remembered that a diagnosis is made on the basis of a simple affirmation by the subject, unlike all other medical diagnoses, which require a battery of supplementary tests in addition to recording symptoms together with the patient's personal and family history. We can therefore safely speak of an "epidemic" of gender dysphoria, but one that has been constructed by manipulating the masses.

Childhood and adolescence are psychologically difficult periods of transition, during which children naturally question their identity, particularly their sexual identity. We've all known a little boy who, for a time, preferred to be a girl and a little girl who acted like a "tomboy" and who, as adults, never pursue these tendencies.
A Canadian study[327], mainly covering a period when

325. Tugaye A., Ernoult E., Vitu V., Schramm S. « Évolution de la prévalence et de l'incidence de la dysphorie de genre en France depuis 2013 à partir des bases médico-administratives ». Santé Publique. 2023; 34(HS2): 145-150. https://pubmed.ncbi.nlm.nih.gov/37336728/
326. Caroline Eliacheff, Céline Masson, *La Fabrique de l'enfant transgenre.* Éditions de l'Observatoire, 2022.
327. "A follow-up Study of Boys with Gender Identity Disorder", Devita Singh1, Susan J. Bradley2, Kenneth J. Zucker2*

pro-trans propaganda did not exist, revealed that the persistence of gender dysphoria in adolescents was very low (12 %), the majority declaring themselves to be homosexual in adulthood. In recent decades, the response to these questions has changed radically. Too many parents no longer dare to say "no" and allow their children to believe that they can get what they want, or become what they think they are, even if this is not feasible, at an age when children are not yet capable of gauging either the reality or lifelong consequences. A section of society and some doctors, out of conformism and/or so-called progressive militancy, encourage them to follow this dangerous path into their future.

Transsexual propaganda is akin to sectarian recruitment mechanisms in its focus on social networks, membership of a community, isolation from family and friends, lobbying, and the rejection of any public debate. Faith is not debatable and those who do not share it must be discredited, ostracised, censored and prosecuted for transphobia.

**The often-violent censorship employed by pro-trans extremists**

Freedom of thought, expression and debate are fundamental human rights and essential elements of democracy. But trans extremists do not see it that way, and accusations of transphobia are a means of intimidation used constantly to prevent any democratic debate (like that of racism or anti-Semitism).

Päivi Räsänen is a Finnish politician who was President of the Christian Democrats from 2004 to 2015 and then Finland's Minister of the Interior between 2011 and 2015. She is being prosecuted by the authorities who accuse her of "*hate speech*", simply because she expressed her ideas on marriage and sexuality in public on a radio programme in 2019 and in a tweet written in 2019 to the leaders of the church to which she belongs. After a unanimous acquittal by the lower court in 2022, the authorities have appealed and seem ready to employ the full legal arsenal in an effort to convict Päivi, as a deterrent perhaps for anyone expressing the same views as her.

"*On the trans issue, we are living in a climate of intellectual terror*", according to Céline Masson and Caroline Eliacheff[328] who warn of the dangers of gender transition for children. Several of their conferences have been cancelled under pressure from trans activists. Numerous calls for demonstrations to prevent them from coming have been posted on social networks by pro-trans associations, ecologists and La France Insoumise, which is in search of constituencies.

A similar experience was faced by the feminist blogger Dora Moutot, who was harassed on social networks[329] then targeted with a complaint filed for "*insults and appeals to transphobic hatred*" after declaring that a

328. https://www.lexpress.fr/idees-et-debats/caroline-eliacheff-celine-masson-l-accusation-de-transphobie-est-une-methode-d-intimidation_2167297.html

329. https://www.lefigaro.fr/story/dora-moutot-feministe-face-a-la-horde-15527

trans woman was born a man, an undisputed biological fact.

Marguerite Stern, former member of the feminist international movement Femen, was the victim of cyber-harassment and an assault, and had to spend time in hospital. Her planned conference in Nantes was cancelled[330] after threats from transgender and LGBTQ+ minority activists.

> "Feminism is in danger, and is more censored than ever. [...] People call me a conspiracy theorist when I say that there's a lot of money coming from the pharmaceutical industry. The industry has every interest in ensuring that this movement flourishes. Those who make the transition become lifelong patients, and those who detransition also have treatments to rebalance their hormonal system ... for life. It's very lucrative. It affects psychologically fragile people, women suffering from post-traumatic stress disorder because they've been subjected to violence and is presented to them as a solution to their suffering… It affects a lot of young people."

Other feminist activists report violence perpetrated by trans extremists: "*We've had eggs thrown in our faces, we've been hit because we hold this position of saying that being a woman is not a feeling, it's a material biological reality.*"

In May 2023, La Part des Anges, a feminist and lesbian bar that had been open for nine years in Rennes city

330. https://www.lemonde.fr/societe/article/2023/04/05/a-nantes-la-venue-de-marguerite-stern-a-un-colloque-annulee-apres-des-menaces_6168322_3224.html

centre, closed after death threats from trans activists who accused its manager of transphobia. The lesbian manager, who campaigns for sexual minorities to have "*the right to go unnoticed*", said she was devastated, financially drained and badly affected by having to let go of her three employees.

During a debate organised by the Centre for Comparative Public Law (CDPC) on "La République universelle à l'épreuve de la transidentité" (the universal republic tested by transidentity), which prompted the Sud Éducation Union to call for its cancellation out of concern for "the transphobic, even racist, violence that some of the speeches might involve", Benjamin Moron-Puech's speech was interrupted[331] [332] by five masked students who sprayed the speakers with paint, stink bombs, marbles and various metal objects, shouting: "*The university belongs to us*" and "*No to transphobes*".

When the British House of Commons debated the Scottish Parliament's Gender Recognition Reform Bill[333], a male Labour MP pointed the finger at a female MP who supported the legal rights of women not to mix with men in changing rooms, toilets and prisons and then crossed the floor of the House to intimi-

331. https://www.lepoint.fr/societe/un-colloque-universitaire-interrompu-par-des-activistes-pro-trans-22-06-2023-2525738_23.php
332. https://www.bvoltaire.fr/des-enseignants-accuses-de-transphobie-agresses-lors-dun-colloque-a-assas/
333. https://www.telegraph.co.uk/politics/2023/01/16/rishi-sunak-blocks-nicola-sturgeons-gender-reforms/

date her more closely. This stand to protect women has been accused of "transphobia" by trans activists.

Meetings of the English feminist organisation Woman's Place[334], which wants to keep certain spaces non-mixed, are still the subject of hostile demonstrations by trans extremists, and the women are forced to meet in secret. Film screenings are stopped by noisy, bearded men dressed as women. Committed feminist professionals are losing their jobs and some are being advised to resort privately to a security agency for saying that biology is a reality.

Sarah Jane Baker was convicted in 1998, under the name Alan Baker, of kidnapping, burglary, unlawful imprisonment and grievous bodily harm with intent. At the Trans Pride March in London, he was cheered when he said: "If you see a TERF [feminist who doesn't recognise trans people as women], punch them in the fucking face"[335]. This is how you find out what "TERFs" are!

Many representatives of sexual minorities, gays, lesbians and trans people, do not recognise themselves in the excesses of trans extremists or those who exploit them. Lio de France, on her blog Double Genre, denounces the weaponisation of trans people:

> "Real trans people are those whose countless difficulties in coming out have transformed them spiritually into peo-

---

334. https://womansplaceuk.org/2018/06/25/references-to-removal-of-single-sex-exemptions/
335. https://womansplaceuk.org/2023/07/10/pride-protest-wpuk-statement-on-london-trans-pride-2023/

> ple open to the world; those who don't want new rights for themselves, selfishly, but for the whole of society. The supporters of the New World Order are using trans people to kick society in the teeth and destabilise it even further.
>
> We trans people want to live in peace and harmony with our partners, our families, our neighbours, our employers or employees, with society as a whole. We don't want to be icons or conned by multinational merchandising services. Making the front page of Time magazine? Big deal, didn't Chancellor Adolf Hitler make it too, having been declared 'Personality of the Year' by the same *Time Magazine* that awarded him the title in 1938?[336]

In Great Britain, certain traditional feminists, renamed Trans-Exclusionary Radical Feminists[337] (TERF)[338], point out that "*there is nothing transphobic about criticising trans ideology; to be transphobic is to discriminate against or incite hatred towards trans people. That's not what we're doing. We're fighting to keep the category of woman indexed to biological sex*", in order to "*effectively combat patriarchy*". J. K. Rowling, herself viewed as a Terf, is being harassed[339] by trans extremists and refuses to bow to "*a movement that I believe is doing demonstrable harm in seeking to erode*

336. https://www.agoravox.fr/tribune-libre/article/les-trans-icones-du-new-business-178621

337. https://www.merriam-webster.com/dictionary/trans-exclusionary%20radical%20feminist

338. https://www.philomag.com/articles/trans-contre-feministes-radicales-la-nouvelle-fracture

339. https://www.lemonde.fr/idees/article/2021/11/26/il-est-ahurissant-d-en-arriver-a-exclure-j-k-rowling-parce-que-ses-propos-derangent-alors-qu-ils-restent-dans-le-cadre-de-la-loi_6103633_3232.html

*'woman' as a political and biological class and offering cover to predators*".

In the USA, the association Gays Against Groomers[340] is a coalition of homosexuals that opposes the recent trend of indoctrinating and sexualising children under the guise of "LGBTQIA+" and denounces the "destructive" practices of certain extremist trans movements that use the LGBTQ+ community as a shield to encourage the "mutilation, sterilization and indoctrination of minors". On 21 February 2023, David Leatherwood, representing this association, explained before the Health and Social Services Committee of the Florida House of Representatives[341] that:

> "For years the LGBT community has fought valiantly for tolerance and acceptance in American society [...]. Now, all our progress is being erased because our community has been hijacked by trans terrorists".

He stressed:

> "The majority of LGBT individuals are against it too [...]. The gay left, in collusion with the gay media and gay advocacy groups [...] are promoting a narrative that the LGBT community supports the medicalization of children, but that is a lie. The LGBT community at large does not support this, it's only fringe radicals."

340. https://www.gaysagainstgroomers.com/about

341. https://lemediaen442.fr/lassociation-gays-against-groomers-accuse-les-militants-trans-de-terrorisme-et-de-promouvoir-la-mutilation-denfants/

**Pro-trans propaganda exacerbates intolerance towards sexual minorities**

Constantly over-reacting to the slightest expression deemed to be transphobic leads opponents to over-react too. The knee-jerk and aggressive activism of pro-trans associations fosters intolerance of sexual minorities, even those who were previously widely accepted. Two sides of the same coin.

In fact, since the spread of pro-trans propaganda, statements, actions, demonstrations and laws against sexual minorities have multiplied in most countries around the world.

In France between 2016 and 2022, anti-LGBTQ+ acts increased by +129 % for crimes and offences and +115 % for infringements. In 2018, the Ministry of the Interior recorded 1,380 homophobic or transphobic offences (an increase of 33 % compared to 2017). In 2019, 1,870 cases: "*This is a gradual upward trend that we have been observing for the past three years.*" In 2022, totalling more than 4,000 incidents, the number of reports rose for transphobic acts in particular, constituting "*the flip side of the propaganda and extremism of some trans people*".

Around the world, pro-trans propaganda is fuelling a backlash and giving rise to laws restricting transgender rights. For example: football players are refusing to wear the T-shirt of the LGBTQ+ ideology that advocates transsexualism and sexual indifferentiation[342].

342. Le Média en 4-4-2.

*La Dépêche* revealed that players Zakaria Aboukhlal, Moussa Diarra and Saïd Hamulic were refusing to wear the shirt. In a statement, the club said:

> "Some players of the professional squad have expressed their disagreement regarding the association of their image with the rainbow colours representing the LGBT movement. Although respecting the individual choices of its players, and after numerous exchanges, Toulouse Football Club has chosen to exclude these players from the match scheduled for this Sunday at 3pm at the Toulouse Stadium. The Toulouse Football Club would like to remind you that 18 nationalities and 5 continents are represented within its professional team. Openness to the world is an integral part of the club's DNA. Our players are chosen for their human qualities, regardless of their beliefs or convictions."

A player's right to freedom of thought is a sensitive issue. Although the club took the decision to exclude those players who refused to wear the rainbow-flocked jersey, it is important to remember that everyone has the right to express their personal convictions. Nantes' Mostafa Mohamed and Guingamp's Donatien Gomis also refused to wear the shirt with the LGBTQ+ colours.

It is a controversy reminiscent of that of footballer Idrissa Gana Gueye, who refused to play in a rainbow-coloured shirt on the International Day Against Homophobia last year. Journalist Bastien Lejeune pointed out the prevailing hypocrisy, namely that at the same time the French

Football Federation was organising the World Cup in Qatar, a country that punishes homosexuality with the death penalty. Facing the onslaught of hysteria spread by some, Bastien Lejeune made a fundamental point:

> "Being homophobic and refusing to endorse or associate with an LGBT ideology that promotes transsexualism and sexual indifferentiation are not the same thing… I think we have the right to disagree and that this injunction is astounding and totalitarian."

In response to the growing trans propaganda, many American States have recently passed laws limiting the derogatory rights of trans people: prohibiting them from having an identity document with a name and sex different from that of their birth, from going to toilets that do not correspond to their birth gender, banning all trans propaganda in schools and prohibiting or refusing coverage by the State of the costs of treatment for sex changes. Arizona passed a law in March 2022 banning surgery to mutilate children struggling with gender confusion[343] and excluding trans women from high-level sporting events.

Utah (USA) has banned these mutilating and dangerous practices by law: the *Transgender Medical Treatments and Procedures Amendments Bill*[344], sponsored by Republican Senator Michael Kennedy, "*prohibits a health care provider from providing a hormonal transgender treatment to*

343. https://edition.cnn.com/2022/03/30/politics/arizona-transgender-health-care-ban-sports-ban/index.html

344. https://www.cbsnews.com/news/utah-transgender-healthcare-spencer-cox-governor-signs-bill-banning-gender-affirming-care/

*new patients who were not diagnosed with gender dysphoria before a certain date*" and "*prohibits performing sex characteristic surgical procedures on a minor for the purpose of effectuating a sex change*".
In Georgia[345], Republican Representative Marjorie Taylor Greene passed a bill prohibiting the provision of puberty blockers, cross-sex hormones and surgery for minors in the name of "gender transition".
In Tennessee, representatives have introduced similar legislation[346] after Republican Governor Bill Lee called for an investigation into a local medical centre that allegedly promoted "transgender" medical procedures for profit.
In Florida[347] and Texas[348] doctors will be prohibited after September 2023 from prescribing hormone-blocking drugs or from performing surgery to modify the sex of anyone under the age of 18.

In Europe, the very states that have pioneered gender theory and transgender transformations have recently severely restricted access to treatments for minors.

In 2021, Sweden decided to block hormone therapy for people under the age of 18[349], except in rare cases. In

345. https://www.npr.org/2023/03/23/1165711935/georgia-bans-most-gender-affirming-care-trans-kids
346. https://www.reuters.com/world/us/tennessee-governor-will-sign-bills-restricting-drag-transgender-youth-treatment-2023-02-28/
347. https://www.reuters.com/world/us/desantis-signs-florida-ban-gender-affirming-treatment-transgender-minors-2023-05-17/
348. https://www.reuters.com/world/us/texas-becomes-largest-state-ban-transgender-care-minors-2023-06-03/
349. https://www.rfi.fr/fr/podcasts/grand-reportage/20211012-la-su%C3%A8de-s-inqui%C3%A8te-de-la-vague-trans-chez-les-jeunes

Great Britain in 2022, the National Health Service decided to close the paediatric department of the Tavistock clinic, which was distributing sex change treatments to minors, following damning reports[350].

In Russia, Parliament has banned the *promotion* of non-traditional sexual relations between young people, and has just banned sex-change surgery[351], except for children with congenital anomalies.

In Singapore[352], magazines are banned from promoting "alternative" lifestyles; *Vogue* magazine's licence to publish has been withdrawn for "*promoting non-traditional families*" and the Prime Minister has announced a forthcoming amendment to the Constitution to "*strengthen the institution of marriage as the union of one man and one woman*"[353].

In Turkey, demonstrations by transsexuals are banned and some demonstrators who have disobeyed the ban have been arrested[354].

---

350. https://www.lavie.fr/actualite/societe/enfants-transgenres-pourquoi-la-clinique-tavistock-va-fermer-en-angleterre-83876.php
351. https://www.theguardian.com/world/2023/jul/24/vladimir-putin-signs-law-banning-gender-changes-in-russia
352. https://www.reuters.com/article/us-singapore-lgbt-heritage-idUSKCN1RC0B6
353. https://www.huffingtonpost.fr/life/article/singapour-l-un-des-pays-les-plus-riches-du-monde-restreint-les-droits-fondamentaux-des-personnes-lgbt_64949.html
354. https://www.reuters.com/world/middle-east/transgender-turks-discrimination-said-loom-larger-2021-07-06/

In Lebanon in 2022, an attempted Gay Pride event was prevented[355] by opponents, the Prime Minister and the Ministry of the Interior ordered the security forces to "*immediately take the necessary measures to prevent any type of celebration, meeting or gathering*" of people from the LGBT community, as "*freedom of expression cannot be invoked in this case, since it is a violation of the habits and traditions of our society, contrary to the principles of monotheistic religions*".

In Africa, trans propaganda has exacerbated intolerance towards this group, with a Ugandan law passed unanimously[356] that placed a penalty of up to ten years' imprisonment on anyone engaging in homosexual acts or claiming to be LGBTQ+.

Cameroon declared persona non grata Jean Marc Berthon[357], who had announced his arrival in Yaoundé following his appointment as French ambassador for the rights of LGBTQ+ people in October 2022. Cameroon's Minister for External Relations, the young Mbella Mbella, recalled at the time that "*the government's position on the issue of defining gender, sexual orientation and sexual*

355. « Liban : Répression illégale contre les rassemblements LGBTI. Annuler immédiatement l'interdiction de rassemblement ; Protéger les personnes LGBTI des attaques ». https://www.hrw.org/news/2022/07/04/lebanon-unlawful-crackdown-lgbti-gatherings

356. https://www.lemonde.fr/afrique/article/2023/05/29/en-ouganda-le-president-promulgue-une-loi-anti-lgbt-accusee-de-violer-de-maniere-flagrante-les-droits-humains_6175301_3212.html

357. https://www.rfi.fr/fr/afrique/20230621-cameroun-yaound%C3%A9-d%C3%A9clare-jean-marc-berthon-ambassadeur-fran%C3%A7ais-de-la-cause-lgbt-persona-non-grata

*identity is clear and not open to debate in Cameroon*" and that the promotion of gender theory "*qualifies as a common law crime*".

Globally, pro-trans propaganda has been followed by a wave of laws sometimes severely restricting the rights of sexual minorities in nearly three-quarters of the world's countries (Africa, the Middle East, Asia, Russia and some European countries).

After decades of relentless lobbying, the reactions are starting to emerge. It is likely that the accelerated spread of propaganda in recent years bears some responsibility now that people's tolerance of pseudo "human rights", the great cloak hiding the reality of all-powerful "merchandising", has reached its limit. Unfortunately, those who are paying the price are the homosexual and even trans minorities who wanted nothing more than to live in peace and quiet, and certainly not be "visible".

# Conclusion

Transsexualism, like transhumanism in general, of which it is a part, is symptomatic of the Western world's disconnection from material reality, and the desire of some people to enter a post-truth, post-human world.
There are physical and biological laws, laws of nature that are beyond our control and that may be frustrating for some of us. But "if bodies, sex, women, or children no longer exist, what is left of the human?"

The road to hell is paved with good intentions. Under the guise of benevolence and inclusiveness, we have ended up celebrating fragile people with psychological problems as role models. Encouraging them along a path that all too often leads to suicide (40 %!) does not help them.
As much as we need to respect the decision of adults who want to change sex, we also need to protect minors *from a trend* (manipulated for political or financial ends) that medicalises them for life, sometimes mutilates them, and

at the very least leads them to a challenging life, fraught with hardship, as chronically ill people.
When adults start to take an active interest in children's sexuality, especially in the classroom, by involving them in practical exercises, is that not simply paedophilia? Since when has it been the role of teachers to initiate children into sexuality? From nursery school onwards?
There is renewed talk of surrogacy in France this coming September, and transhumanists would love nothing more than the few children permitted to live to be conceived *in vitro*. Politicians looking for electoral votes are rushing to support them with a draft law (La France Insoumise party).
In short, its supporters want transsexuality as the new norm, gender theory as the new orthodoxy, and treatments dispensed without the advice of doctors (an endangered species). For this to become the norm, it must be repeatedly suggested as a possible variant of sexual identity.

**Counter-revolution versus *cancel culture*[358]**

The "*counter-revolutionary*" strategy proposed by Christopher Rufo is an example of the thinking that is taking place in many circles and individuals.
According to Rufo, the great vulnerability of the American cultural revolution lies in the fact that it lives on a drip-feed of public funding. The most urgent task for its opponents is to expose the nature of the ideology, the way it operates, and put together a plan to fight back and

358. Bring on the Counterrevolution - Christopher F. Rufo (christopherrufo.com)

abolish it through a democratic process.[359] A political programme proposed by Rufo is to subject the current regime to simple tests: have living conditions improved or deteriorated? Are cities safer? Can children read?
A good idea that could be applied in France, where leaders for forty years at least have been repeating the same tested techniques that have led to the organised failure of education, research, the suburbs (apart from a few chosen individuals sheltered in selected schools such as the Légion of d'honneur), and so forth.
He said and wrote that instead of liberating the black militant from his inferiority complex and his despair, the racial revolution has driven him into this psychological state. Critical theorists, who claim to represent the oppressed, are in fact nothing more than a bureaucratic class fully protected from the constraints of the private sector. They think they're organic intellectuals à la Gramsci when they're really just paper tigers. Professors at Harvard, Columbia and UCLA are not warriors. They don't threaten the system, they depend on it.

The same applies to our academics, one such case being Sandrine Rousseau, the famous "ecologist" and now deputy for the NUPES coalition party. A Lille University professor?
Given the copy-and-paste nature of our leaders (behind America by about 10 years) and the accelerating influence of American choices via the omnipresence of consultancy firms (McKinsey, etc.) who dictate their decisions to our

359. Christopher F. Rufo, *America's Cultural Revolution: How the Radical Left Conquered Everything* (Broadside Books, 2023), 352 p.

rulers, an analysis of the means available to people to regain power in the USA can be instructive to the French and Europeans more broadly, the European Union being no more than Biden's puppet. For Christopher Rufo, the counter-revolution must begin by restoring meaning to the basic desires of Americans. It must be a positive force aimed at restoring what has been demolished. To achieve this, it must lay siege to institutions that have lost the public's trust. Its aim is not to control the bureaucratic apparatus but to break it down.

That's the crux of the matter, particularly in the field of medicine where the Regional Health Agencies, the armed wing of the government, have managed to shatter what was one of the world's leading healthcare systems at the turn of this century.

The example set by medicine can be applied to university teaching, medical research, theatre, the arts and so on. Anyone hoping for public funding has to choose a fashionable subject.

> "The counterrevolution must take its bearings from the common citizen and offer to restore his dignity and mastery over his own life. It must reverse the process of institutional capture, break up centralized ideological powers, and return influence to local communities.
>
> For decades, conservatives in Congress have effectively written a blank check to captured institutions, experienced dismay at the subsequent behavior of those institutions, and then continued to fund them. These are all policy choices – and they can be changed. On the first day in office, the new president could prepare executive

> orders targeting the concepts and formulations that have traveled from the fringes of the 1960s Left to the center of American power. At the head of this list would be a ban on the government promotion of left-wing racialist ideology, or critical race theory, and to abolish the "diversity, equity, and inclusion" bureaucracy that serves as its administrative vehicle. The order would replace all this with a system of strict color-blind equality, prioritizing the values of equal treatment, individual excellence, and race-neutral decision-making. As part of this policy, the president could also rescind Lyndon Johnson's Executive Order 11246, which established the legal basis for "affirmative action" – a euphemism for state-sanctioned racial discrimination in the interest of favored identity groups – and forbid the use of identity-based quotas, preferences, and "disparate impact" analysis as an acceptable basis for any federal decision-making, to the fullest extent of the law."

The counter-revolution must arm the population with a set of values, expressed in a language that goes beyond today's ideological euphemisms, and restore a healthier sense of history that inspires rather than shames. The deepest conflict is not one of class, race or identity, but between elite institutions and ordinary citizens. The counter-revolution must enlighten the latter about the nihilism that threatens to bury them and contribute to restoring the role of the executive, the legislature and the judiciary to the exclusion of the social engineering that is rampant nowadays.

**Towards the abolition of the WHO? [360] [361]**
Shouldn't the politicians responsible to the electorate be looking together at the need for a complete overhaul of the international non-governmental organisations that are partly State-financed, such as the WHO, the UN, NATO and all their institutional offshoots that consider themselves to be the real powers and treat the people with contempt?[362]

The injunctions on children's health care and sex education that the WHO[363], through its unelected leaders, is seeking to impose, should rouse us to reject them wholesale. We must not rely solely on the countries that dismiss Western supremacy to get rid of these increasingly totalitarian organisations, but free ourselves from the subservience shown by the majority of people in the West during the pandemic. As Dr Thomas Binder says: "Enough is enough".[364]

When, in France, will we see an opposition worthy of the name: courageous and selfless, finally putting France's general interest above all other considerations? Until those happy days arrive, parents are the only ones who

360. *Nouveau Monde.* « Un groupe international d'avocats s'oppose à la prise de pouvoir de l'OMS » (nouveau-monde.ca)
361. Nouveau Monde. « La transformation de l'OMS en dictature hygiénique » (nouveau-monde.ca)
362. *Nouveau Monde.* « La députée européenne Christine Anderson contre l'OMS et les milliardaires misanthropes » (nouveau-monde.ca)
363. Must-see video by J.-D. Michel relating to this article: *Nouveau Monde* — « OMS: vers un putsch mondial?! » (nouveau-monde.ca)
364. Dr. Thomas Binder Interview - How Psychology Was Weaponized To Suppress Truth In The Age Of COVID | Children's Health Defense Europe (childrenshealthdefense.eu)

can protect their children from school-related harm. Pauline Quillon concludes her book with a few simple suggestions:

> "What can be done by parents to avoid this madness, and how can disorders be dealt with and reduced if they occur in their child? The answers are astonishingly simple, given the scale of the evil phenomenon described here; they can be summed up in a few words: educate your child, listen to him, talk to him, be vigilant (shows, smartphones, friends), provide him with role models who will turn him away from narcissistic self-absorption and lift his soul".

# Annexes

1. Reproduction of Table 34 in Alfred McKinsey's book *Sexual Behavior in the Human Male* (1948).

| AGE | NO. OF ORGASMS | TIME INVOLVED | AGE | NO. OF ORGASMS | TIME INVOLVED |
|---|---|---|---|---|---|
| 5 mon. | 3 | ? | 11 yr. | 11 | 1 hr. |
| 11 mon. | 10 | 1 hr. | 11 yr. | 19 | 1 hr. |
| 11 mon. | 14 | 38 min. | 12 yr. | 7 | 3 hr. |
| 2 yr. | 7 | 9 min. | 12 yr. | 3 | 3 min. |
| | 11 | 65 min. | | 9 | 2 hr. |
| 2½ yr. | 4 | 2 min. | 12 yr. | 12 | 2 hr. |
| 4 yr. | 6 | 5 min. | 12 yr. | 15 | 1 hr. |
| 4 yr. | 17 | 10 hr. | 13 yr. | 7 | 24 min. |
| 4 yr. | 26 | 24 hr. | 13 yr. | 8 | 2½ hr. |
| 7 yr. | 7 | 3 hr. | 13 yr. | 9 | 8 hr. |
| 8 yr. | 8 | 2 hr. | | 3 | 70 sec. |
| 9 yr. | 7 | 68 min. | 13 yr. | 11 | 8 hr. |
| 10 yr. | 9 | 52 min. | | 26 | 24 hr. |
| 10 yr. | 14 | 24 hr. | 14 yr. | 11 | 4 hr. |

**Table 34. Examples of multiple orgasm in pre-adolescent males**

Some instances of higher frequencies.

2. Full version of the text sent to rectors for academic affairs (2021)

For several years now, the Ministry of Education, Youth and Sport has been committed to combating homophobia and transphobia by raising awareness throughout the educational community of the effects of violence based on sexual orientation and gender identity, and by preventing such violence. This commitment is part of an interministerial initiative, coordinated by the Interministerial Delegation to Combat Racism, Anti-Semitism and Anti-LGBT Hate (Dilcrah), whose roadmap is the National Action Plan for Equal Rights and Against Anti-LGBT Hate and Discrimination 2020-2023 [1].

Its chapter entitled "Promoting inclusive education and overcoming prejudice" calls, in particular, for special attention to be paid to transgender students or students questioning their gender identity [2], taking into account their situation and that of their families.

As a public service founded on the principles of neutrality and equality, schools have a duty to welcome all pupils in all their diversity and to ensure the integration of each of them, with the aim of enabling them to succeed in their studies. It promotes respect for others. It is based on the values of the Republic and therefore on a universalism that defines each person not by their identity but by their dignity as a human being. Schools should not create special rights for this or that category of pupils, but they should offer each of them, beyond their personal trajectories, an environment conducive to their success at school, which is the primary aim of our institution.

Transidentity is a fact that concerns schools. Like families, schools are confronted with situations where children - sometimes as early as primary school - or teenagers are questioning their gender identity. In practical terms, while each situation is unique, in the case of children and teenagers this often takes the form of a series of actions aimed at socially affirming their gender identity, such as changing the way they dress and/or asking to be referred to by a new first name. It can also lead to psychological distress and, in some cases, harassment.

Staff may understandably be unsettled by these requests and, in any event, are faced with highly practical questions relating, for example, to the use of a chosen first name or of private spaces, the answers to which are currently patchy and often improvised. This can create situations that are detrimental to the well-being and therefore the academic success of the pupils concerned. They can also cause difficulty for some staff, or even expose them to liability risks.

This circular relates exclusively to the school context and is not intended to deal with the whole issue of transgender minors or minors questioning their gender identity - for the sake of simplicity, hereinafter referred to mainly as "transgender pupils". This text is aimed at all staff, whether they work in primary or secondary education, its purpose being to remind them, in accordance with common law, of the rules to be followed when dealing with transgender pupils, and to share the best practice implemented in schools to better support and protect such pupils, regardless of their personal development paths.

It is vital that we all work together to create school environments that guarantee these pupils their right to integrity, wellbeing, health and safety. It is therefore essential that each member of the educational teams is able to understand the needs expressed by the young people concerned, to protect them by putting in place individual support measures that have necessarily been developed in conjunction with the families, and also to deploy general and preventive measures guaranteeing each pupil the best possible chances of personal fulfilment, perseverance and success at school, which is the primary aim of our institution.

1. Understanding the realities and the diversity of transidentity situations

Support for transgender children and teenagers or those questioning their gender identity can be hampered by the persistence of preconceived ideas about transidentity and a lack of knowledge about their backgrounds and rights. Knowing and understanding the issues surrounding gender identity and the realities of the lives of young transgender people is a prerequisite for taking proper account of these pupils in a school setting.

Health institutions, in particular the World Health Organisation (WHO), recognise that incongruence between gender at birth and experienced gender is neither a psychiatric disorder nor a pathology. Gender identity is in fact unique to each individual and his or her personal experience.

In this respect, the European Court of Human Rights notes that the concept of "private life" mentioned in Article 8 of the European Convention for the Protection of Human Rights and Fundamental Freedoms (ECHR) "includes not only a person's physical and psychological integrity, but can sometimes also embrace aspects of an individual's physical and social identity. Elements such as gender identity or identification, names, sexual orientation and sexual life fall within the personal sphere protected by Article 8 of the Convention" (ECHR, 6 July 2017, Case of A.P., Garçon and Nicot v. France, nos. 79885/12, 52471/13 and 52596/13, paragraph 92).

In practice, this means that consideration of a pupil's claimed gender identity must not be conditional on the production of a medical certificate or diagnosis, nor on the requirement of an appointment with a health worker.

Transgender people have rights under international, European and French law. Subject to certain conditions, they may obtain changes to their civil status, independently of any physical transition or medical procedure. However, only adults and emancipated minors can obtain a change of gender in their civil status.

Transgender people are also protected. Transphobic acts and language are punishable by law [3]. Furthermore, the fundamental right to privacy set out in article 9 of the Civil Code rules out any disclosure of a person's transidentity without their consent.

Finally, it is important to bear in mind that each situation is unique. Student questioning of their gender identity does not necessarily lead to a transition process. They must be listened to attentively and sympathetically so that their free choice is respected while care is taken not to create an irreversible situation that would be in breach of this freedom.

The student's journey may often go through stages of social affirmation (change in appearance or not, adopting a preferred name or not), voluntary disclosure of gender identity (or "coming out") to friends, family and school, before eventually leading - or not - to administrative procedures (changes to civil status) and/or medical procedures (these are by no means compulsory in a transidentitary journey). In all cases, the school must be careful to ensure that the conditions are in place for an assertive transition - i.e. the possibility of being and remaining identified and visible as a transgender person - or a confidential transition.

These young people are by no means a homogeneous population. Their journeys are not always linear and can follow very different timelines, alternating periods of questioning, action and pauses. Each person is free to continue, stop or resume their transition pathway. Teachers have a duty to support young people and to show them the greatest compassion, to give them the opportunity to explore a variety of paths without stigmatising them or locking them into one path or another.

2. Knowing how to respond to the circumstances of transgender students

Given the diversity of these situations, all support measures put in place for young people who are transgender or questioning their gender identity must be designed individually on the basis of the needs expressed by the pupils and their families, whilst respecting the rules common to the school establishment. They are based on three principles :

- Listening ;
- Supporting ;
- Safeguarding.

a) Listening to students and their families : accommodating the questions and needs of young transgender people
In many situations, pupils and their families together approach the education team with questions about the possibilities of transition in the school environment and the practical conditions for supporting the pupil. The first guiding principle then is to listen actively and sympathetically to the questions and needs expressed by the pupil. First and foremost, students need adults

to acknowledge their reality and their concerns. This means being attentive to their specific requests and lived experiences and reassuring them that it is legitimate to ask questions. Listening respectfully and giving students the opportunity to express themselves, without prejudging their needs, helps to create a relationship based on trust and support.

It is also important to remember that certain issues affecting the student's privacy - relating to their body or medical history, for example - need not be discussed unless the initiative to do so is taken by the student.

At the same time, it is essential to reassure the family who will be supporting the pupil during the process that the school is able to protect him or her and put in place proper arrangements for learning. The pupil, his/her legal representatives and the educational team can then work together to identify the best support measures to ensure the pupil's wellbeing at school.

If a pupil alone raises the issue of his or her gender identity with a member of the school staff, communication with the legal representatives should only take place with the pupil's explicit consent. Respecting this principle of confidentiality is vital: in some cases, unwanted disclosure of a young person's transidentity may expose them to a serious risk of rejection or violence.

Conversely, if requested by a pupil, the educational team has a duty to create the conditions for constructive dialogue, or even mediation, with the legal representatives, in an effort to seek a consensus and encourage better consideration of the minor's circumstances.

In cases where a minor appears to be in danger within the family or living environment, a decision may be made to record and pass on worrying information to CRIP (French unit for the collection of information of concern) or to file an official report with the prosecutor's office for children.

b) Supporting a transgender pupil: implementing personalised measures to support and protect students
The foremost responsibility of the staff of a school or educational establishment towards a transgender student is to protect his or her health, safety and right to an education. This means taking concerted action with the pupil and his or her legal representatives. In many cases, enabling a transgender student to make the transition under the right conditions means that students who have been withdrawn from school can return to school.

**First name changes**
For the pupils concerned, adopting a new first name and requesting the use of pronouns corresponding to their gender identity can be very important steps. It should be noted that minors may, with the consent of their legal representatives, request a change of first name in the civil registry [4], but that the use of a preferred name is a necessary step before any change in civil status. For many young transgender people of school age, social rec-

ognition of their gender identity is achieved by using a preferred name.

Most commonly, when a minor's civil status has not been changed, if the application is made with the consent of both parents [5], the aim is to ensure that the chosen first name is used by all members of the school community, as respect for a pupil's gender identity should not be left to the discretion of adults and other pupils [6].

Similarly, the school will support this change by substituting the preferred name, consistently and simultaneously, in all documents relating to its internal organisation (roll-call lists, school lunch card, library card, etc.) as well as in digital workspaces, etc. Conversely, the fact that continuous assessment is used in examinations for certain national diplomas means that the pupil's first name entered in the civil status register is alone considered in the information systems that monitor student grades [7].

Despite the school's commitment to supporting the pupil, it cannot however make such changes without the consent of the legal representatives. The exercise of parental authority, which covers a set of rights and duties in the interests of the child, cannot be called into question.

> Article 371-1 of the French Civil Code: Parental authority is a set of rights and duties whose ultimate aim is the interests of the child. It is vested in the parents until the child reaches the age of majority or is emancipated, in order to protect the child's safety, health and morality, to

> ensure the child's education and to enable the child's development, with due respect for the child's person. Parental authority is exercised without physical or psychological violence. Parents shall involve their children in decisions that concern them, taking into account their age and degree of maturity.

For example, if the parents of a pupil under 18 years of age object to the use of a preferred name requested by their child at school, it would be in the pupil's best interests to initiate a dialogue with his or her family.

In the rare event that a change of civil status has been obtained, all administrative documents relating to the pupil's schooling and examinations must be rectified as soon as possible to bring them into line with the identity documents. At the person's request, diplomas and school reports issued with the old first name must be reissued with the correct first name.

**Gender expression and dress codes**

In addition to the use of first names and preferred pronouns, respect for choices relating to clothing and appearance is also an important aspect of recognising the gender identity of these young people. It is the responsibility of staff to ensure that pupils' gender expression is not questioned or mocked, particularly by other pupils and staff. The measures adopted to combat harassment and cyberbullying in the pHARe Programme (to combat harassment at school) apply particularly to this type of situation.

It is also important to ensure that school rules, particularly those relating to dress, are not subject to gender-specific instructions. For example, permitted and banned clothing and accessories apply to all pupils without distinction, particularly when these bans are justified by safety requirements. The same applies to the wearing of make-up and jewellery - including on vocational courses and during periods of on-the-job training.

**Use of private spaces**

The pupils concerned may also express worries about the use of private areas (toilets, changing rooms, dormitories) where there are no appropriate facilities (e.g. mixed toilets). At the request of the people concerned and depending on the availability of facilities, various options may be considered:

- Where possible, the school may allow the student access to individual toilets and private areas in the changing rooms and within the boarding school;
- The school may permit the pupil to use the toilets and changing rooms in accordance with his or her gender identity, taking care to deal with the situation when the pupil concerned is identified by his or her peers as being transgender;
- The school may permit the pupil to occupy a room in a part of the boarding school that conforms to his/her gender identity under the same conditions; a solution may be sought in consultation with the fellow pupils of the pupil concerned for the sharing of a room; in any event, the solutions implemented must necessarily be consensual;

- The school may agree with the pupil to set up flexible hours for the use of changing rooms and communal bathrooms/showers.

Particular care should be taken in these areas, where all students, and especially young transgender students, feel more vulnerable and are more particularly exposed to the risks of violence and harassment.

As far as possible, the choices made regarding toilets, changing rooms and dormitories should also apply to school trips and outings. With the permission of the pupil and his/her legal representatives, schools may need to contact - for example, in the case of an external sports competition or a school exchange - another school or host site to ensure that the pupil has access to safe facilities that meet his/her needs.

c) Protecting transgender students against all forms of discrimination, harassment and violence

Like all students with vulnerabilities, transgender students are particularly exposed to the risks of harassment and cyberbullying. They are also frequently the victims of transphobic comments and violence from pupils and adults in schools. It is the role of the educational team to protect them. School staff, particularly school health staff, must be able to identify and respond to such behaviour and the suffering it causes. In order to deal more effectively with this type of behaviour, schools can implement preventive measures as well as provide support for victims and hold accountable and punish the perpetrators.

Given the risk of transgender pupils or pupils with questions about their gender identity dropping out of school, staff at the school or college will also look out for signs of unease or any downward trend in school performance. Failure to take account of a pupil's transidentity can quickly lead to the development of school phobia and a drop-out scenario.

As with all pupils, the educational team is also attentive to the health of these young people and will ensure that they have access to in-house consultations provided by child and adolescent professionals trained in these issues. Particular attention must be paid to the appearance of co-occurring disorders (anxiety disorders, depression, suicidal risk, substance abuse, self-directed aggression, etc.), which are more common in young transgender people than in the general population.

Most of the time, the support measures put in place to accommodate transgender pupils do not raise any particular constraints or difficulties for the school. They are all the easier to put in place if they have been planned in advance and the school policy and internal rules explicitly take into account the needs of the young people concerned.

3. Preventing transphobia: introducing general preventive measures

Finally, the inclusion of transgender pupils or pupils questioning their gender identity can only be achieved if every school, college and lycée strives to create a caring environment for all, whether transgender pupils are enrolled there or not, most notably by zero tolerance for transphobic abuse. This policy of preventing transphobia must be part of a collective, cross-disciplinary approach and part of the fight against all forms of gender-based violence and discrimination.

**A collective, partnership-based approach**

This collective approach is led by the school's management. It plays a central role in informing staff (in some situations, managing information also means respecting confidentiality and privacy) and coordinating the educational team. It is up to the school to remind staff of their responsibility to support and protect these pupils. Ensuring that they are treated with respect also means that the adults in the school must be aware of the issues surrounding gender identity. The presence of trained staff who are able to listen to pupils' views in a safe environment and support them individually and, where appropriate, their families, contributes to this approach. Training sessions are regularly included in the national training plan and in educational training plans. Depending on the specific context of a school, the head of the school may also decide to adapt his or her policy on preventing transphobia and supporting young transgender people by setting up a local training initiative.

Each education authority has resource persons who can be mobilised, namely gender equality officers (see directory), LGBT+phobia observatories, sex education advisors, social workers and harassment referral teams within the local education office, under the widespread roll-out of the pHARe harassment prevention programme. They can be called upon for training and educational projects in schools, and to identify local community partners. In lower and upper secondary schools, the gender equality officers can be key contacts.

This policy must necessarily be part of a partnership approach and draw on all the available expertise (professionals working with children and young people, educationalists, social and health workers, etc.) and on the support of associations approved or accredited by the national education authorities, which help to raise awareness among pupils and provide staff training. Parent representatives should also be involved.

**An integrated, cross-disciplinary school policy**

Action taken by the school will achieve the set objectives if it is part of a coherent policy to combat all forms of gender-based violence. Policies to prevent transphobia are all the more effective if they are combined with efforts to combat sexism and homophobia, while paying attention to the specific nature of transphobic violence.

It also requires a number of tools to be deployed as part of the school's policy :

- Consider the administrative and material implications of expressing the diversity of gender identities.
Example: Put in place a process to facilitate the replacement or addition of a preferred name in internal administration documents.

- Prevent violence between peers
Example: Include the specific features of gender-based and LGBT+phobic violence in the harassment prevention policy, organise awareness-raising initiatives, build on sex education projects.

- Develop educational initiatives
Example: 17 May, International Day Against Homophobia and Transphobia, is a date on the calendar for educational initiatives. Each year, it provides an opportunity to mark an important moment for recognition and reflection on issues relating to sexual orientation and transidentity.

- Encourage and promote support practices between students
Example: Support student initiatives to prevent gender discrimination and violence (discussion groups, student council activities, etc.).

- Develop transphobia prevention through learning situations
Example: Ensure the delivery of content relating to transphobia in the curriculum.

4. Resources

Tools and resources relating to the prevention of homophobia and transphobia and to support for LGBT+ pupils are available on the Eduscol website, in the dedicated area "Preventing LGBTphobia": https://eduscol.education.fr/1590/prevention-des-lgbtphobies?menu_id=1956

The Minister for National Education, Youth and Sport, Jean-Michel Blanquer.

---

[1] The acronym "LGBT" stands for "lesbian, gay, bi, trans". The + sign is added to include all people whose sexual orientation and/or gender identity deviate from the dominant norm.

[2] A transgender, transidentitary or trans person is someone who does not identify with the gender of their birth. This includes anyone who has made or wishes to make the choice to transition, whether socially, administratively, legally or medically.

[3] See articles 225-1 and 132-77 of the Criminal Code, relating to discrimination and aggravating circumstances in crimes and offences respectively.

[4] Minors, however, cannot change their gender in civil status records using the procedures set out in article 60 of the French Civil Code.

[5] Students of legal age or emancipated minors can decide alone on the administrative changes that concern them.

[6] In his general recommendation of June 2020 on the

rights of transgender people, the French Human Rights Defender, in a case brought by a transgender secondary school pupil who was confronted with the teaching team's refusal to take his gender identity into account, ruled that "any act related to gender identity suffered by a person [...] and having the purpose or effect of violating his or her dignity or creating an intimidating, hostile, degrading, humiliating or offensive environment" constitutes prohibited discrimination within the meaning of the Act of 27 May 2008.

[7] School management applications will gradually be adapted to allow for these changes.

[8] The school climate survey conducted by the French Evaluation, Forecasting and Performance Department (DEPP) among secondary school students in 2017-2018 highlighted the prevalence of homophobic violence. The survey on the health of LGBT people, led by Arnaud Alessandrin and Johanna Dagorn, the results of which were published in 2020, found that 72 % of young trans and/or non-binary people described their school experience as "bad" or "very bad". The survey carried out in 2018 by Gabrielle Richard for MAG Jeunes LGBT, with the support of Unesco, also showed that two-thirds of young trans people report having been targeted by verbal violence from their peers at school and around one-fifth by physical violence[365].

---

365. Source: Education.gouv.fr

## Thanks

Thanks to the translators Anne, Elin and Isabelle, for their efficiency, their precision and their kindness and availability, and to the Michalon-Fauves team, which is always available to provide citizens with medical information that is usually difficult to find.

Thank you to all the parents and grandparents, the whole family and friends who watch over the future generation by protecting them from psychological aggression.

Thank you to numerous volunteers in France and other countries, who help us and others to transmit the message!

## Table des matières

www.ingramcontent.com/pod-product-compliance
Lightning Source LLC
LaVergne TN
LVHW010917051026
849532LV00003B/724
*9791030205183*